Dedication

This book is lovingly dedicated to my friend Jo,
who inspired me by her courage and compassion.

With special gratitude to Dennis, Jo's husband,
for the support and encouragement to write this book.

And to all of Jo's family, friends and caregivers
who loved and supported her on this journey.

FOREWORD

I am delighted to write this foreword for Rose Simon because she has written a book that provides valuable resources for stroke survivors and their caregivers. *Jo's Journey - A Resource Book for Stroke Survivors, Caregivers and Coaches*, not only emphasizes the importance of an at-home recovery program but it also shares the ups and downs of my wife's journey to recovery and the cognitive gains that she made.

There is a strong need for the information in this book. Stroke patients who are discharged from hospital or rehabilitation facilities are dependent on out-patient rehabilitation programs to receive the therapy exercises they need for recovery. Unfortunately, even the best insurance policies will cover only a certain amount of therapy visits. After insurance benefits end, the need for cognitive and physical rehabilitation still exists. It is up to the stroke survivor and their family to pay for caregivers or rely on family and friends for assistance. So many people do not know where to begin. I suggest beginning with *Jo's Journey*. There are many good books on the subject of stroke to read and I encourage you to learn all you can. This is one of the good books and it will give you plenty of helpful and practical information that you can use right away.

Life changed dramatically for my wife and I when Jo woke up with a severe headache many years ago. Unfortunately, her stroke was at first mis-diagnosed and many valuable hours were lost. When she finally underwent surgery, which was supposed to be two hours, but ended up being ten hours, she was left in a coma for four-months. The doctors gave her a three to five percent chance to live. However, I wasn't ready to give up. I read everything I could about stroke and stroke recovery. I was encouraged to learn that current neuroscience research has found that the brain can continue to learn and repair itself beyond the traditionally held belief of a six-month window. This is referred to as neuroplasticity.

All the research indicated that focused and repetitive activities and exercises are necessary for rebuilding connections in the brain. Unfortunately, it takes time and dedication to sift through all the resources available. As my wife's primary caregiver, I had very little extra time to come up with stimulating exercises. It was about a year after my wife's stroke that I realized I needed more help. I hired Rose to work with Jo on her speech drills and to do some gentle hand exercises and stretches with her. It was not long before Rose began suggesting other activities beyond speech drills to help my wife improve her thinking skills.

I was very impressed with Rose's suggestions for activities that were simple, easy and that made sense. As a former engineer, definable goals and measurable results are of paramount importance to me. The activities and exercises Rose used clearly showed which thinking skills she was targeting, and how she was measuring progress. She explained to me the various activities she was using with Jo and what rehabilitation goals were being targeted. I was impressed at the changes I saw in my wife's ability to control a pen and paintbrush with her left hand. When I heard Jo play a tune by memory on the piano, I knew Rose was definitely on to something. What made that activity so impressive was that Rose had never played the piano before but had found an easy way to teach both Jo and herself. I could see the positive effects the activities had on Jo when I came in the room after their sessions and saw her smiling and laughing. Jo usually didn't want to stop painting and it was exciting to see her focus her attention on her work. When I looked at her paintings, I couldn't help recalling when the doctors had told me she only a three to five percent chance of survival. Jo had come a long way!

If you are looking for new ideas and activities to help improve communication and thinking skills after stroke, *Jo's Journey* will provide you with the resources. The activities in this book, along with the extensive speech exercises, will help you put together an effective at-home cognitive training program as well as support any existing rehabilitation therapies.

Dennis Dille

JILL,
I WANT TO THANK
YOU FOR EVERYTHING
YOU DID TO HELP JO NOT
RECOVER. WE COULD NOT
HAVE MADE THE PROGRESS
WE MADE WITHOUT YOU. THANK
YOU MY FRIEND FOREVER

Denny

CONTENTS

INTRODUCTION

This is a story about one woman's amazing journey towards cognitive recovery after a life-altering stroke–and the strides she made when we used the creative arts to revive a host of cognitive functions. I was fortunate to be Jo's traveling companion on this journey that began with squiggly line drawings, and evolved into painting whimsical birds. Together we explored the world of music, which helped her improve her memory, as we learned new songs on the keyboard and tapped out rhythms on the drum. We also spent time reading and writing stories and poems. To an outside observer, it might have seemed like we were just having a lot of fun, and we were, but less apparent was the monumental challenge of learning and re-learning that Jo undertook to improve her thinking (cognitive) skills.

Everyone has their own way of learning and does so at their own speed. What works for one person might not work for another. According to Howard Gardner's Multiple Intelligences Theory (MIT), outlined in his book, *Frames of Mind*, people have innate preferences for the way they learn and process information. These preferences indicate what areas of intelligence are most active in an individual. There are eight documented intelligences that have been shown to be localized in specific regions of the brain. They are linguistic, logical-mathematic, musical, spatial (art), interpersonal (ability to understand others), intrapersonal, (the ability to understand oneself), naturalist (ability to learn from the natural world), and spiritual. Gardner's theory has been used by educators and applied to research on stroke victims suffering from aphasia at Boston University and with children at Harvard's Project Zero.

When I began working with Jo, I chose activities that appealed to several of her intelligences at once to get all areas of her brain activated. At least that was my hope. The art activities involved spatial-art and kinesthetic learning, and sometimes, intrapersonal learning. Music activities involved kinesthetic, linguistic, mathematical, interpersonal and obviously, the musical intelligence. Storytelling and writing involved the linguistic, interpersonal, intrapersonal, kinesthetic and even spiritual intelligences. This MIT theory informed the foundation of my master's degree in Interdisciplinary Arts and Education from the University of Montana. This teacher's program also encouraged the use of critical and creative thinking processes to create meaningful learning experiences. We learned how to create lesson plans, measure progress, make assessments, and design learning experiences. This education would prove invaluable in my work with Jo.

As long as I can remember I've been fascinated by how the brain learns and retains new information. When I was a young mother looking for ideas on how to prepare my son for preschool, I came across a book that would change my way of thinking about thinking. *Seven Kinds of Smart* addressed seven of Gardner's eight intelligences. The ideas in this book had a profound effect on me—and kickstarted my curiosity in this direction. It was fascinating to consider that intelligence could be multifaceted. From the moment I discovered these ideas, and years later when I studied Howard Gardner's book in graduate school, I started to see the value in incorporating this theory into teaching situations. While MIT theory may still be gaining broad awareness and acceptance, most of us are familiar with the three learning styles: visual, auditory and tactile. Visual learners prefer pictures, diagrams or symbols. A person who prefers learning "hands on" is a tactile or kinesthetic learner. Auditory learners prefer to take in information by listening. With all that in mind, I decided to put together a "program" that would incorporate Multiple Intelligences Theory, the different learning styles and the use of the creative arts for cognitive exercises.

Before we began working together, I had had no previous experience in caregiving or coaching (beyond raising two children and several years of substitute teaching). My background was in college admissions, and program development for several non-profit organizations. Although I did not have coaching experience specifically, I led *Journal to the Self* ® writing workshops written and developed by Kay Adams, (LPC, RPT), a leading theorist in the field of journal therapy. As a certified instructor, I taught these and other writing workshops to women's groups, especially cancer survivors as well as at colleges and in community venues for over two decades.

Even so, nothing had prepared me for working with a stroke survivor. I believe my lack of experience was an advantage because it put me in the beginner's mind, without any preconceptions or hard and fast rules. I was willing to experiment and test out new approaches and ideas. I tested them out on myself first to be sure I understood and could explain the steps simply. Then I observed whether or not they were effective on Jo. The success we achieved together provided the impetus for sharing this story.

Looking back, I believe it was a very serendipitous meeting when Jo's husband asked me if I had ever done caregiving, to which I answered "No." However, I surprised myself by saying that I would consider it. Those words opened the door to what would be a fascinating eleven-year coaching relationship which culminated with the writing of this book. The first time I met Jo she was sitting in her wheelchair, next to her husband. Not knowing what to expect, I was nervous, but Jo quickly put me at ease with her lopsided, but welcoming, grin. I remember thinking at the time that despite her challenges, she had such a gracious spirit.

I liked her instantly. I think we both intuitively knew that we would end up working together. Neither of us had any idea what to expect.

In one way, it was easy to work with Jo. She put her all into doing her best every day. She never complained about the tedious speech and swallowing drills or the other activities that challenged her. After a year of consistent effort and practice, when Jo was still struggling with vocal sounds, she said to me, "I'm sorry. I hope you don't grow tired of me." It was pretty much at that moment I knew I was in for the long haul. I did not want to leave this amazing woman just as she was beginning to show some signs of improvement. Yet, working with Jo's physical and cognitive limitations was anything but easy. Each gave us many challenges to overcome. I had the challenge of developing exercises that Jo could do with her limited memory and understanding. I had to make my directions easy to understand. I also had to adapt the drawing, keyboarding, and other exercises to accommodate her use of only one hand, her weak, non-dominant hand. Most of all, we both had to work through the daily challenge of communicating our thoughts and words so we could understand one another.

The exercises in this book were developed after months of trial and error—and Jo's forward and backward progress. Not every activity we tried worked, but I have presented the ones that did. I found that some of the best ideas were common sense exercises with an element of fun tossed in. When selecting particular ones within the areas of speech, writing, art, music, and storytelling, I focused on targeting as many of the thinking skills as possible. Some of our activities were real cognitive workouts, like playing the piano. Since I knew nothing about playing a piano or keyboard, I was learning along with Jo and feeling the challenge!

Jo taught me many things during our years together. I think the most important one was that hope can come from hopelessness, and courage can arise out of fear. Jo was one of the most courageous people I have ever met. Unfortunately, she did not believe that about herself. Every time she struggled past one hurdle or climbed another mountain, she revealed her boundless courage. Jo had good reason to be scared of the momentous journey she faced. It was no small feat. There were times when she thought she couldn't do it anymore. She was afraid she would not improve; afraid she would not find herself again. And yet, Jo showed up every day to do what she needed to.

Jo spent her life offering hope to others through her service work and her general approach to life. She would have liked to have known that her journey to recovery might benefit other people who are facing monumental challenges. Jo has been an inspiration to me throughout our journey together, especially during the last days of her life. She taught me that when it comes to recovery, each day is a new day, and brings new hope. It was an honor for me to have spent time with Jo, whose grace, compassion, and courage continues to inspire. She demonstrated what each of us could accomplish when faced with incredible hardship and challenges.

✳

The information presented here is from a creative art and not a medical perspective. The suggested activities in this book are designed as a launching pad for your own creative ideas. The exercises can be used over and over again. It's the not quantity of exercises that is important, but the quality. The questions provided after many of the exercises, can be used to encourage your client's feedback on the activities. Your client's answers can guide you towards simplifying or increasing the cognitive or physical challenge of each.

THIS BOOK HAS TWO SECTIONS.

Part I describes Jo's journey to recovery and what happened when specific exercises were used to strengthen her cognitive skills. Basic information on stroke recovery, types of therapy, and rehabilitation expectations, along with guidelines for hiring caregivers and coaches are included. There is a section with suggestions for dealing with caregiver burnout and negative emotions. In the chapter Goals and Objectives, several tools are offered to help you measure your loved one's or client's progress and to set learning goals.

Part II provides exercises that target the cognitive domains of attention, memory, visual processing, language, and executive function. A large section of the book is devoted to improving speech and communication. These exercises can support an existing speech therapy program with facial exercises, voicing drills, and language building exercises. The activities are easy to follow. It is the most substantial part of the book and the one I refer to the most.

When it comes to the creative arts, you can start anywhere. Naturally, it makes sense to start with the ones that your loved one or client has interest in or experience. Art, music, writing, and storytelling each have a dedicated chapter. The exercises can be made simple or complex depending upon ability. Although not everything in this book will work for everyone, I am confident you will find plenty of exercises or ideas that will.

To all those on the journey of recovery and those assisting them, I wish you the best. I hope that this book can provide you with practical information to make your journey easier. The most important thing to take away from reading this book is that consistent cognitive training using the creative arts, can improve attention and memory skills at the minimum. As one improves in these areas, the creative arts can stimulate the cognitive functions of decision-making, problem-solving, reasoning and even self-reflection.

Part 1

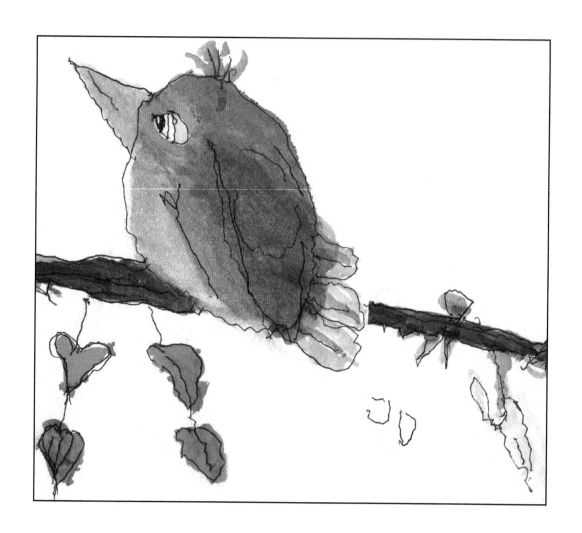

Becoming again like they were in the beginning.

—JoAnne

CHAPTER ONE

JO'S JOURNEY

I am on the path few take. —JoAnne

JoAnne, or Jo for short, was a petite, dark-haired woman with smiling eyes, a warm smile and a quick sense of humor. Before her stroke, she had been an active professional in health and human services where she developed health and safety programs for hundreds of employees. In the span of her career, she was the director of health and human services for three large health care systems. Jo's compassionate nature made a difference in the well-being of others every day. It must have been very difficult for her, a person who had helped so many people, to suddenly need help herself.

Jo's stroke damaged her left hemisphere which controls speech, comprehension, arithmetic, language, and the motor functions of the right side of the body. The damage left her struggling to communicate. The muscles that controlled her speech (jaw, lips and tongue, soft palate, and vocal cords) were not functioning correctly. She had lost the ability to pronounce sounds correctly and to speak at an average volume and pace. It was difficult for others to understand her, and the simplest words were a struggle for her.

The stroke took away a big chunk of Jo's memory. It left her struggling to remember people's names, what day it was, and the events of yesterday. She had great difficulty remembering words. It was hard for her to repeat back short phrases or spell words. Learning new information and retaining it was a great challenge for her. Her thinking processes had been affected by the stroke, including her ability to reason, problem-solve, and make decisions. Jo described her condition like this, "The more I think of something, the more difficult it is to remember. When I am not thinking, it is easier."

Jo had many physical challenges to face after her stroke. It took three months, with the help of a tilt table, for Jo to be able to be vertical and maintain her blood pressure and respiration in that position. She dealt with frequent urinary tract infections, headaches, bladder infections, and bouts with pneumonia. She had an internal catheter and a tracheostomy tube in her throat to help clean and remove secretions from her airway and to deliver more oxygen to her lungs. Her nutrition came through a feeding tube. Jo's right side of her body was weak and immobile. Her right hand was clenched into a hard fist, and her fingers remained tightly contracted. Despite years of massage and exercise, her right hand never became functional again. She had to train her non-dominant hand to do everything. This hand was subject to jerky, involuntary movements and it was hard for her to reach and grasp.

Jo's physical therapy regime consisted of bending and stretching the weak muscles of her right leg and arm. Since she had balance issues, she could only stand for a few moments while holding on to something or someone. Unable to walk by herself, she struggled with her walking exercises. She had great difficulty with them, and her pain increased when she walked. She needed assistance from her bed to the wheelchair. She was unable to raise her body upright, turn over and swing her legs over the edge of the bed. When I asked Jo how she felt about her walking, she said, "Everything is out front. I don't see my feet out in front. Hard to see. Afraid to see them and walk. Lots to remember. I can't get it in good time."

To complicate things further, Jo had vision problems that were not able to be resolved. She described it as, "everything is moving." It affected her balance and probably contributed to her fear of falling. After many visits to eye doctors, changes in prescriptions, eye exercises, and even cataract surgery, Jo's vision continued to trouble her. It challenged both of us for every activity we did. We used magnifying lamps, large typewriter keys, stickers, and other adaptive devices.

Jo faced a momentous uphill path to recovery. It required all her focus, determination, and courage to keep going. It was heartbreaking to watch her struggle with the most basic of mental and physical tasks that most of us take for granted.

Before her stroke, Jo had enjoyed cooking gourmet meals, entertaining, and remodeling her home. She took great pride in her beautiful waterfront home and looked forward to spending time traveling with her husband in retirement. Jo had a master's degree in public health and managed essential career responsibilities. She worked with lots of people and made many decisions daily. Now, post-stroke, she found herself semi-isolated in her home, unable to move independently, unable to remember one day to the next and having to be reminded how to swallow correctly.

Jo's husband, Dennis, believed that his wife could get better, maybe even walk someday. The stroke had put an abrupt end to their retirement dreams, leaving them both shocked and helpless at the magnitude of its damage. Jo's husband was an incredible advocate for his wife. He would not give up hope. He read books on stroke rehabilitation and the different therapies available. He was not afraid to ask questions of the medical professionals or to change doctors if he felt they were not satisfactory. He became quite proficient at all aspects of caretaking, but it was more than one person could handle.

Dennis decided to put together an "A" team, as he called it, of medical professionals to help in his wife's recovery. I was the only non-medical support person. The rehabilitation team included a physical therapist, a speech therapist, and a medical doctor at the time. My role on the team would be the at-home coach helping her with speech exercises assigned by the speech-language pathologist. The therapist gave me specific rehab goals to work on, which included swallowing, volume, diction, and speech practice. The physical therapist gave me exercises for Jo's hands to help her recover strength and control. Other than a few exercise handouts from these therapists, there was no roadmap for the cognitive recovery part of the journey. After several months of following the speech pathologists' exercises, I showed the therapist some of the new activities that Jo and I had started doing in our sessions. She was impressed with the additions and gave me the green light to use them. That encouraged me to continue to add more exercises that might "boost" the cognitive homework up a notch, providing novelty in the learning process for Jo.

Starting from our first session together, I was learning how fast Jo could process information and what she could remember. Each day was different, and I varied our activities to her abilities. It was not hard to make adaptations. Even small changes often made a difference. I started our sessions off by observing Jo's attention and her ability to understand and follow directions. I also asked her how she was feeling and if she had any pain. That information helped guide me in selecting activities she would be able to do that day. It also showed me how discomfort or pain could influence cognitive abilities and performance. I was beginning to understand how suffering pain could affect thinking skills.

After several months of getting to know each other, Jo opened up and began to talk about her recovery and her feelings. She told me how hard it was for her to do the things she had to do. She often spoke about her fear of falling. Whenever the subject came up, I would stress the importance of having patience with herself. Once she told me, "People don't know what I am trying to accomplish. I am on the path few take." Unfortunately, Jo would equate her self-worth with her ability to walk. "It's miserable," she said when explaining her walking practice. She said that she just wanted "to walk and be one with myself."

When these feelings of despair arose, we would watch videos about other stroke survivors. She asked me if they were also afraid. "What did they do to face their fears?" Jo also expressed concern about not being able to do anything right. She asked me why it was taking her so long to improve. Jo could not remember her successes and would quickly lose patience with herself. On those days when she said, "I can't do anything right," we talked about climbing mountains—one step at a time—and staying focused on her goals. She told me that she enjoyed hearing those words and said that she needed to listen to them often.

Birds held a particular fascination for Jo and her husband; they brought her joy. That is the reason why they were a subject of her artwork. Dennis kept their many birdfeeders flowing, and all kinds of birds came to their porch to feed. Jo and her husband would spend time outside on their porch while they watched the doves, sparrows, and other songbirds visiting the feeders. It was a peaceful activity for her.

Jo once told me,

> The best part about the weekend was watching the birds. They were waiting for me to arrive. It felt very peaceful.

Another time she said,

> Becoming again like they were in the beginning. The birds are part of this. It would be sad if there were no birds. Birds like to hear us. We keep them company. We sound good to them.

I tried to find other activities that would bring Jo joy or peace and help relieve her depression. We listened to all types of music, watched funny videos, and sat outside and watched the sun sparkle on the water. Jo often told me how much she enjoyed our quiet moments together. However, there was so much to do during our sessions, that finding Jo time for merely "being" with herself was a challenge. Using guided imagery exercises helped to give her that quiet time and they also helped to manage her pain.

FOCUSING ON THE COGNITIVE DOMAINS

The following are the five cognitive domains that Jo and I focused on each day.

- Attention
- Memory
- Language & Communication
- Visual Processing
- Executive Function

ATTENTION

There are five types of attention: focused, sustained, selective, alternating, and divided.

At the beginning of our first year together, Jo's attention span was less than a few minutes. Sometimes this was due to discomfort, illness, or difficulty focusing. She would often forget what she was doing in the middle of an activity and would need directions repeated several times. To assist her, I kept all distractions to a minimum, gave simple instructions, and repeated them often. I also gave her time to rest between activities.

When Jo demonstrated an ability to do so, we began working on exercises that required sustained attention. We did reading and story-telling exercises, drawing, and some math exercises. During our sessions, I would remind Jo to pay attention to her head and body posture and to notice if she was drooling. She did not seem to be aware of what her body was doing when she was concentrating on something else. It was difficult for her to do two things at once.

Over time, Jo showed improved attention and memory skills by playing games and following simple directions. By our fourth year together, Jo had demonstrated improvement in three levels of attention: focus, sustained, and selective. She could complete a 20-minute keyboard typing exercise, watch a 90-minute movie, and remember piano notes. Jo came along way from the place she began, only being able to focus for a few minutes. Now she was able to be aware, attentive, and engaged in exercises for a sustained time. It was exciting to witness this improvement! There were even a few occasions where she could work alone on activities without constant supervision or requests for repeated directions.

MEMORY DOMAIN
Memory is the ability to recall and retain information.

Jo had difficulty remembering what happened the day before and even that morning. She mentioned that whenever she went to sleep, she would forget everything that just happened. She had great difficulty repeating and concentrating on tasks, but by the end of the first year, she was concentrating for about four minutes without asking for directions. Repetitive mathematical and word exercises, recall questions, journal writing, and music were some of the activities I used to help her strengthen her short-term recall skills.

After six months, Jo began to use the computer keyboard to type. She also showed progress in writing words and thoughts in her hand-written journal. During the year, I added more speech and language exercises like multisyllabic word drills, sentence-building activities, spelling, and alphabetizing. We continued to focus on retrieving words and naming objects and colors. Over time, she went from calling all the colors "yellow," to naming eight colors correctly.

Whenever I could, I tried to connect the current activity to another activity in her past to help trigger memories. Jo loved to cook and travel, so we watched cooking and traveling shows and talked about them. We might supplement the activity by drawing something related to the topic. We practiced implicit memory skills or the ability to do things by rote. We practiced recalling the days of the week, months of the year, seasons, and counting by fives or tens. We sang familiar Christmas carols. She did better remembering phrases that had a sing-song rhythm to the words. It was important that whatever new information I introduced to her, held some meaning to her. She needed to be motivated to remember it because the task of remembering was so tremendous for Jo.

Again, the progress was not linear and often challenging to understand. Some days Jo could recall information with over 75% accuracy and other days not so well. The activities of writing and music helped her improve her memory. When Jo first began writing, she repeated the same word or phrase several times and needed a writing prompt to get her going. Over time, she improved to where she could sit and type without a prompt and express what was on her mind. Although there was still a repetition of thoughts and sentences, it was getting less frequent. Her spelling had also significantly improved!

Over the years, Jo's memory skills continued to improve, and by the third year, she was able to play several short melodies and two complete songs on the piano without prompts or looking at the sheet music. She knew where all the notes were and could name some of them. By the fifth year, Jo was playing three new piano songs. She was also learning how to use the keys on the computer keyboard like backspace, delete and how to close the dialogue box when it popped up.

LANGUAGE & COMMUNICATION
The ability to use language and communicate thoughts and words.

Jo's speech challenges remained a constant factor throughout the years I worked with her. Some days were better than other days. Jo and I would begin our speech sessions with facial massage and lip, tongue, and mouth exercises. Jo's face and jaw were tight, which caused her to have her mouth open all the time. Each day we worked on breath control, swallowing, volume, pitch, vocal rhythm, and all aspects of speech. Swallowing was always hard for Jo, and she might make ten attempts before she could swallow. It was hard to understand her words and impossible to decipher between the close sounds of "B, P, D, or T." She could not speak three words in a row because she would run out of breath or forget what she was saying.

By the second year, Jo's speech had improved, but she continued to lose air from her trach hole, which made it hard to understand her. During this time, we used a voice wave machine to target individual sounds so Jo could hear her voice. Jo needed practice on volume, consonant distinction as well as speaking sentences in a regular, rhythmical pattern. Her tongue, which flopped to one side, was showing some improvement. At this time, the speech therapist instructed me to skip over the beginning tongue and lip exercises after she had shown improvement. We were to continue with the facial and mouth exercises. Around this time, I introduced scribing in our activities. Jo would speak, and I would scribe her words. It was a prolonged and challenging process with lots of pauses. I would repeat back her words and go over each word to be sure I had heard her correctly. Afterward, we would read her words on the computer screen and make corrections. She was very good at pointing out typos!

By the third year, Jo's speech had improved with the removal of her trach and her vocal cord procedure. Her breathing capacity had greatly improved; she could hold a sound for 18-20 seconds. Although Jo still needed reminders to swallow, clear her throat, and speak louder. Swallowing remained a constant challenge for Jo for the rest of her life. Sometimes, Jo shared her frustration about her condition. She told me that her "mouth leaked" or "got tired" after speaking one sentence. One time she pointed to her cheek and said, I don't talk a lot because of the hard work involved. The fluid in my mouth has gotten worse." She commented that swallowing was an "artificial thing to do. When I asked her to explain, she said, I have to take my time to think it through. I don't remember having this problem before. I wish I didn't have this problem.

Jo's language skills showed definite improvement over the years. Eventually, she was able to retrieve more words and articulate them. Together we wrote several short stories about the birds she had painted. She also showed increased self-awareness. When I asked her to tell me what was her heart's desires, she said the following:

I want to accomplish things by myself, to know the desires of others, and to help them achieve it.

To be more giving and say the right words to others.

To be a better giver.

To have more strength and more knowledge to do the right thing.

To be healthy and free from pain.

To be balanced and able to hold myself well.

To stand up for myself and others.

VISUAL PROCESSING DOMAIN

Visual processing or visual-spatial skills is the ability to interpret information from our eyes. It is the ability to understand the shape, size, color, and orientation of objects.

Art exercises opened a new world for Jo. When we began, Jo had difficulty understanding the edges of shapes. Vision difficulties might have been affecting her success. Eventually, she was able to do drawings from an example or image provided. We started with pastel chalk because it was comfortable to hold, and she could feel the connection between her fingers, chalk, and the paper. Jo learned how to blend the chalk colors. Her first two drawings were of a sunflower and a sunset, both pleasing.

By the third year, Jo had progressed extraordinarily well with art activities. She was drawing or painting several days a week, and her concentration and skill level had improved substantially along with her fine motor skills. She could paint thick and thin lines and hold her paintbrush at different angles to achieve desired results. For the next several years, Jo became more proficient at drawing and painting, mixing colors, choosing colors, and composition. Jo continued to show fantastic improvement in this area and painted over 50 watercolor images and sketches. Some of her watercolor paintings were on display at a local gallery, which brought her a great sense of accomplishment and pride.

EXECUTIVE FUNCTION DOMAIN

Executive functions include self-awareness, goal setting, self-initiation, planning, organizing, self-monitoring, self-evaluation, flexible thinking, problem -solving, and metacognition.

We did not practice the executive thinking skills until Jo's attention, comprehension, and memory skills improved. These cognitive skills were higher-level skills and the fact that Jo was able to achieve them with some success, was terrific! We began by working on sorting objects, categorizing objects, and doing matching and sequencing activities. We did simple math, puzzle, games, and handwriting practice using second and third-grade language and math workbooks. I timed these exercises to help gauge her progress.

This cognitive work was arduous for Jo in the early years. She had difficulty comprehending and completing the activity in a reasonable amount of time. However, with daily practice, Jo showed cognitive gains. She showed interest in advanced exercises like reading and discussing essays and poetry. Jo also showed improvement in communicating her thoughts and feelings through her writing and storytelling. She sent emails to family members, and she loved reading their emails back to her.

We focused on her ability to problem solve in all our activities. I wanted Jo to figure out how to help herself when she was stuck on a problem rather than say, "I don't know." The underlying goal behind all the exercises I used was to help her reason and problem solve. In the beginning years, these were distant goals, but over time, they slowly started to happen in increments. Art activities, in particular, required the higher-level thinking skills of reasoning, decision making, self-assessment, and self-correction.

TOWARDS THE END OF OUR JOURNEY

During the last two years of Jo's life, she developed cancer and gradually started to lose some of the cognitive and motor abilities that she had gained over time. We had to make many adjustments to our activities to reflect her current abilities. This part of her journey started to mirror the beginning of it as Jo began to lose her ability to focus, follow directions, and, sadly, even remember her name.

Jo's speech had declined to just a word or two. She was having such difficulty swallowing that she needed a food peg for her nutrition. Pain and illness were taking a significant toll on her ability to concentrate and perform the same activities that she had accomplished during the first nine years of her recovery. She also showed a marked decline in both her gross motor skills as well as fine motor skills, and her walking exercises ended. Jo's left hand became more rigid, and she could not hold a pencil properly anymore, which affected her ability to draw.

For art activities, we returned to the first exercises of drawing lines and shapes. Jo had great difficulty replicating bird and human forms. Even when we used examples of her previous artwork to show what she had been able to do, her ability to draw began to decline. I decided to try collage and watercolor exercises again. Fortunately, with some assistance, Jo was able to paint four abstract watercolor angels two months before she died. It was the last exercise that she showed interest in and was able to complete.

Watching short videos and listening to music were the activities that replaced the more cognitively challenging exercises of previous years. Jo could no longer play on the keyboard with her left hand because she was unable to spread her fingers across the keys. Jo's attention and focus had declined, and she would forget what she was doing in the middle of the activity. Often, she would sit in her wheelchair with her head drooped to one side unaware or not caring about what was going on around her. Knowing that this decline in her abilities distressed her, I made sure not to make that much of it. I instead tried to find things that would make her smile or bring her pleasure. Whenever possible, I made a big deal of her achievements, no matter how small.

During the last weeks of her life, JoAnne grew less and responsive until our sessions became bedside visits. We watched several movies together. The last two films were her favorite ones: *Charade* with Audrey Hepburn and *The Wizard of Oz*. It had become an effort for Jo to keep her eyes open, but she did for those movies. We also looked at beautiful books with paintings of birds and nature. I read her favorite poems and stories while she lay still but awake. I played music that I knew she would like, including "Somewhere over the Rainbow" and "The Nutcracker Suite," as well as soft piano and flute music.

Jo's daughter and son visited during her last week of life. Jo's eyes lit up when she saw them walk in the bedroom. It was amazing to see her spirit revived. I believe that was the most joyous gift that Jo could have ever received. They snuggled next to her in bed as they read Dr. Seuss books to her--the same ones that she used to read to them as children. She smiled when they gave her a yellow stuffed puppy. Perhaps the love Jo had for her family and others gave her strength and courage during her final days.

Jo left this world with grace, gentleness, and compassion, just as she had lived her life. I am forever indebted to her for the things she taught me on our journey together. Every day she showed me that even when faced with terrible loss and hardship, each day offers an opportunity for hope and improvement.

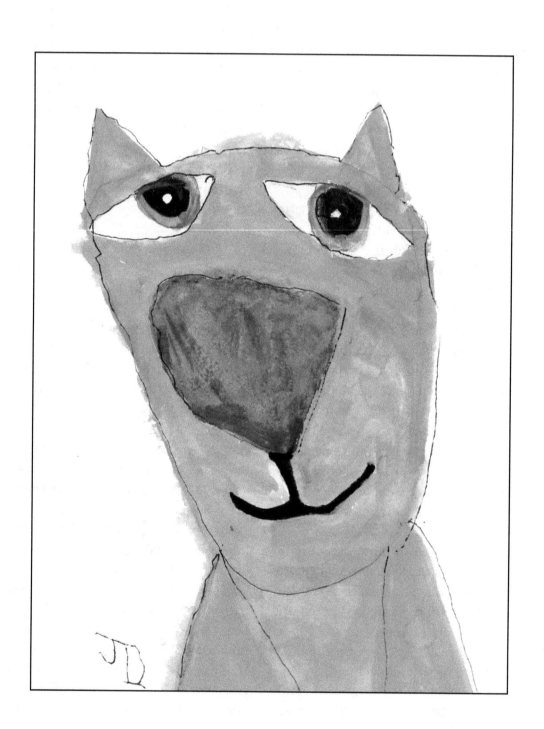

CHAPTER TWO

EMOTIONS AFTER STROKE

The best way to begin this topic is by sharing Jo's own words when she was feeling low in spirits:

I don't have a memory.
There is nothing in me worth finding.
All I know is what someone tells me.
I can't do anything right.

DEPRESSION

It is essential to know that depression can appear anytime post-stroke and can disrupt the recovery process significantly. Many stroke survivors will experience moments of depression that range from low self-esteem to deep despair. For some, these moments seem insurmountable and endless. Stroke survivors need the opportunity to talk with a licensed counselor or participate in a stroke support group. Communicating with others who have experienced a stroke is very helpful for understanding what to expect during recovery. If stroke survivors don't have an opportunity to discuss their feelings, they will feel they are on the path few take.

Family members and caregivers can provide needed encouragement, but that is not always enough. The stroke patient needs to see how other stroke patients are coping in their recovery. They need to be able to talk and interact with each other. I discovered how important this was when I read books to Jo about other stroke survivors. She was engaged and asked many questions. Sometimes she expressed sadness at her situation. When this happened, I gave her an opportunity to let out her emotions without interference or judgment. I felt at a loss for finding the right words and knowing the techniques that a trained counselor might use. I just had to do the best I could as a compassionate human being. Sometimes, I did not feel I was doing enough. The magnitude of her grief, which she hid most of the time, was overwhelming when she shared it. Sometimes I was speechless, even tearful. Sometimes all I could do was hold her hand and let her know that I supported her.

I am not a professional counselor, and there are techniques and approaches that a counselor might use that would be more effective. Many stroke survivors worry about the extra burden they may be putting on a family member, who is often their primary caregiver. They might have difficulty expressing this as well as handling the emotions of grief and guilt that may surface. With a professional counselor, the patient can feel free to talk more openly.

Here is an example of a type of *talk therapy*. I would ask these questions whenever Jo expressed a negative opinion about herself, such as "There is nothing in me worth finding."

TALK THERAPY QUESTIONS:

- What makes you say that particular thing?

- Do you think others think or feel that way about you?

- Can you remember a time when you did not think that way about yourself?

- How would you feel if you did not think that way about yourself?

- Would you like to hear about some positive things that I know about you?

I would talk to Jo about being more compassionate and patient with herself. She had been a nurse for decades and a loving mother. I would ask her if she would think such negative thoughts about her children or her patients. She always answered that she would not. I explained that she deserved to give the same compassion and patience to herself as she would others. I would tell her about some positive traits about herself or the accomplishments she had made until I saw subtle changes in her expression. Sometimes she would ask, "Do you mean that? Am I like that?" Then I showed her drawings that she had made, stories she had written, and other accomplishments she had done. Unfortunately, she could not remember how much progress she had made over the years and needed constant reminders that she was improving. Luckily, I kept examples of her early work and could show her the difference.

Often, during these low-spirited times, I would introduce an activity that I knew she enjoyed or would make her laugh like watching "I Love Lucy" episodes. I also put on silly animal videos showing cats and dogs doing funny things. Sometimes, I turned down the lights and put on a guided meditation tape. Other times, I encouraged her to lay back, close her eyes and listen to some beautiful classical music while I gave her a head massage. Most of the time, these activities helped change her attitude.

How can you help those suffering from low self-esteem and depression?

First, recognize and respect the stroke patient's feelings and let them know you are listening to them. Be encouraging, but do not set over-enthusiastic expectations. Instead, talk about what is most likely to happen and celebrate accomplishments. Let the survivor know that the recovery process can be long and slow, and that healing is individual. Some other suggestions:

- Find ways for the stroke survivor to connect with other stroke survivors through support groups, both in-person and online.

- Talk with health professionals about professional counseling services.

- Reconnect with family members and friends.

- Go out on outings and to community events. Do not wait for total recovery to begin enjoying life again.

- Be sure to incorporate a fun activity whenever possible.

- Research vitamins and food supplements to enrich the diet.

- Play soothing music in the home and during sessions.

- Watch funny shows, read humorous stories, and laugh as often as possible together!

- Make time for relaxation. Not every moment needs to be devoted to rehabilitation.

In conclusion, I would like to say that I saw how the harmful effects of depression could affect a person's ability to learn and do activities. On the days when Jo was depressed, she completed her exercises slower than usual, her concentration was weak, and she complained about her pain more. One of the many valuable lessons I learned from Jo was that depression has severe effects on our brain. Our ability to concentrate, problem-solve, and remember can be affected. Depression can also affect our body, our immune system, sleep patterns, digestion, and our ability to handle pain.

FEAR

Everything is upside down. Everything is out of sync. —Jo.

Jo often brought up issues about her fears. She was sad by how much the stroke had ravaged her mind and body, leaving her searching for her "old self." She feared she had lost her sense of identity. She also had fears that she might not recover or that she was not doing things right. Yet, the biggest concern of all was her fear of falling, and we spent hours discussing that fear and trying to figure out ways to handle it.

So many times, I wished I had a magic wand that could take away her fears. I believed her fear interfered with her success in walking. How could it not? Even with assistance in walking, she could not let go of her fear of falling. When she practiced walking, she was not thinking about the mechanics of walking, but instead, she was thinking about falling. Fear of falling is a common fear in stroke patients and others who have suffered a traumatic brain injury. If a stroke patient falls, their fear of falling again increases. Because of this fear, they might further restrict their activity or movement, which, unfortunately, only compounds the situation. Less movement equals poor motor skills. It is a vicious cycle. Caregivers and family members must understand how powerful this fear of falling can be and not mistake it for lack of motivation.

In our discussions about her fear of falling, I would ask Jo, "What makes you the most fearful about falling?" I thought that was a good place to start. I wanted to know what caused the fear to surface. Was it during the transfer process from chair to feet or the initial steps of walking? One answer Jo gave was:

It is difficult to see my feet because of my back and head position. Everything is out front. Don't know what my feet are doing. I think I am doing things right. Don't see my feet out in front. Hard to see. Afraid to see and walk. Lots to remember to do. I can't get it in good time.

One suggestion for managing fear of falling is to ask your client or family member what would make them feel more confident when walking. A stroke patient must be involved in this most important exercise. They also need to know that you recognize this fear of falling as valid. Here are some common sense things you can do to assist the stroke survivor as they learn to walk again.

- Avoid uneven surfaces or stairways, and remove obstacles like rugs and furniture when walking.

- Use prescribed walkers and canes to help offer support.

- Keep all verbal distractions and background sounds to a minimum.

- Walk on a comfortable surface.

- Wear good supportive shoes.

- Walk at a comfortable rate of speed. Avoid going faster than one's comfort or ability level.

- Check for vision or balance issues.

Here are some suggestions for you to consider using with your family member or client to help you both understand the fear of falling. Do not forget to speak about these concerns with a medical practitioner!

- First, ask these two essential questions: What would make you feel safe? What makes you feel unsafe?

- Allow the survivor to express their fears in a safe, nonjudgmental atmosphere and give them support.

- Watch videos, read inspirational books, and have discussions on how other people have overcome fear and physical limitations.

- Consider adding a licensed professional counselor might to join the recovery team for a while.

- Treat the anxiety with compassion and understanding, which will help the stroke patient work his or her way through it.

- Learn more about how the fear of falling can impact recovery.

WHY JOY IS SO IMPORTANT

The most wasted of all days is one without laughter. —E. E. Cummings

Joy can turn things around and help us get through difficult times. Research tells us that joyful people have less chance of having a heart attack. They have healthier blood pressure, lower cholesterol, controlled weight management, and decreased stress levels. It may be because happy people tend to exercise, eat healthy foods, sleep better, and avoid unhealthy habits. Most of us know the importance of taking making time for pleasure every day. It is not something you wait for tomorrow or the next day to begin. Laughter makes us feel good. Laughter also has some positive health benefits. A hearty laugh is like a mild workout; it gets the blood flowing, and releases endorphins, which are natural painkillers and mood boosters.

As I have mentioned before, Jo consistently demonstrated that emotions and cognition are closely related. Whenever her spirits were down, so were her cognitive abilities. Attitude affected almost everything we did in our sessions, even down to handwriting! I added more "joy producing" activities when she felt low-spirited. We played games, watched comedies, listened to opera and classical music, and watched movies. Since, I wanted to know what particular things made Jo happy, I asked her to do the following exercise.

ACTIVITY: Create a Joy List

This pleasant exercise involves thinking about what revitalizes, restores, and recharges you. Take some time to list the things, people, and activities that make you happy and which ones you would like to have more of in your life.

1. What makes you happy?

2. What makes you curious?

3. List activities that you enjoyed doing alone before your stroke.

4. List activities that you enjoyed doing with your spouse or other people.

5. Pick five joyful things that you could add to your life right now.

Try not to hurry through this exercise. Let it be an enjoyable experience allowing for pleasant memories to surface. When your loved one or client is finished writing or dictating, go over the lists and discuss them by asking the following questions:

1. Which of these activities, if any, are you doing now?

2. Which ones are you not?

3. What is the reason these activities are not happening?

4. Are there new activities that you would like to do with your spouse, friend, family member, or just yourself?

5. What changes or adaptations need to occur to bring back these activities or parts of these activities to your life?

ACTIVITY: Watch "Feel Good" Movies, Musicals or Comedies

Jo and I watched movies to exercise attention, memory and communication skills. After about 15 to 20 minutes into a film I would pause it. We would then do a small recap of what was happening in the movie. We did this several times throughout the movie. This exercise required a tremendous effort on Jo's part to remember the story and then talk about it. Even though Jo continued to have great difficulty accessing words and verbalizing, I could tell when Jo understood the movie. She answered my simple questions and showed appropriate emotions. In selecting films, look for positive themes that can offer inspiration or lightheartedness. Always ask your client what they would like to watch.

MINDFULNESS

When we are in the present moment, we become more grounded in the world around us and more centered in our selves. When this happens, we often become aware of what we never noticed before---but what was always

there. We become more aware of our bodies and our breath. We gain a greater sense of peace and acceptance when we are present to ourselves. Here are some mindfulness activities that Jo enjoyed while sitting outside, observing the natural world.

ACTIVITY: Attentive Listening

For this exercise, listen to some peaceful music with your client. Be sure they are in a relaxed position. Encourage your client to let the music flow over and through them. Ask them to listen to the individual sounds of the instruments and experience the music for what it is. For this exercise, the music is all that exists. After the listening session is over, encourage your client to talk or write about this experience. Here are some questions you can ask:

1. What did you experience during this time of attentive listening?

2. What thoughts came in your mind?

3. How did the music make you feel?

4. What was this experience like for you?

ACTIVITY: Practicing Awareness

For this activity, sit with your client in a peaceful setting for five or ten minutes to observe and experience their surroundings. Encourage your client to practice attentive seeing, listening, and conscious breathing. If your client has difficulty, remind them that they can pull themselves back to the present moment by focusing on their breath. After the awareness activity is over, encourage your client to review it by asking them the following questions:

1. What did you observe?
2. What did you see?
3. What did you hear?

4. What did you feel?

5. What thoughts flowed into your mind?

Be free of judgment and expectation, and just let whatever happens happen. There is no goal here other than to be in the moment. You are not looking for a specific experience – you are allowing whatever comes up to come up.

WAYS TO HAVE MORE JOY AND LAUGHTER IN YOUR LIFE

- SMILE.

- Do something you love every day!

- Surround yourself with things that give you pleasure.

- Look for the humor in everyday situations.

- Read jokes and humorous stories.

- Watch comedies, movies and TV shows

- Spend time with light-hearted people.

- Spend time with children who love to laugh and do silly things.

- Enjoy time with an animal or pet.

- Listen to music that gives you pleasure.

- Allow some creative expression into your life.

- Stay connected with family and loved ones.

- Exercise and eat nutritious foods.

- Be compassionate to yourself and others.

- Avoid negative emotions.

- Avoid negative people.

- Begin a gratitude journal.

- Practice mindfulness.

- SMILE.

ALWAYS CELEBRATE SUCCESSES ALONG THE WAY!

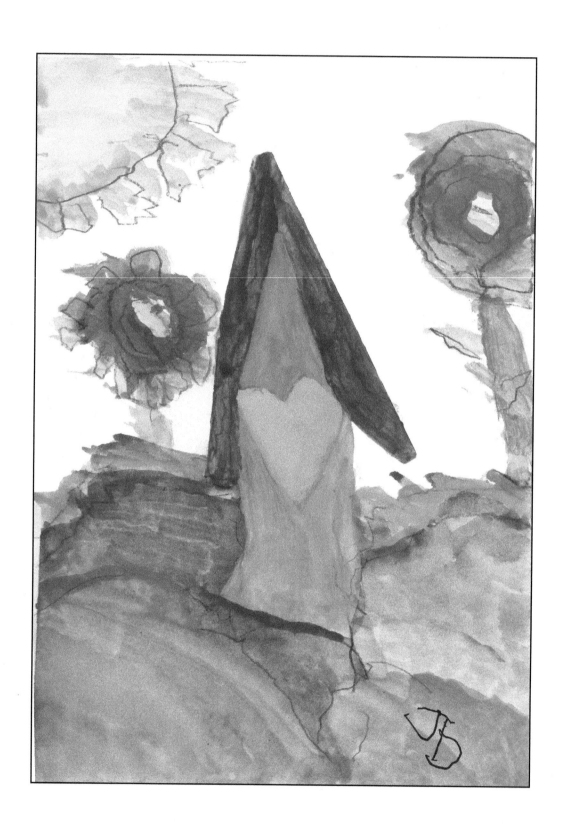

CHAPTER THREE

CAREGIVING

Caregiving can take a physical, mental, and emotional toll on the primary caregiver, which is usually a family member. The responsibility can be overwhelming, especially during the early days of recovery when the stroke patient comes home. The primary caregiver may find that they are responsible for round the clock care and have little idea of how to manage it all. There are doctor appointments, activities of daily living (eating, bathing and dressing), meals, shopping, house, and yard maintenance, and social and family obligations. It is exhausting.

As a family caregiver, you may be realizing that the life you shared with your loved one has taken a drastic turn, and it may never be what it was before the stroke. You may never be able to share the same activities the same way, or you may never hear your name spoken from your loved one's mouth. Family caregivers may find that they are becoming more of a parent or coach than a spouse. Especially difficult is when the survivor was the primary income producer or homemaker in the relationship. Not only has a stroke affected the survivor with a variety of symptoms, but it has also removed them from their primary role in the household.

Often both the family caregiver and the stroke survivor opt-out of social engagements for a variety of reasons. It takes energy and planning to accomplish these outings. There also might be a certain amount of embarrassment, fear, or anxiety in facing new situations or the reactions of others. Through it all, the element of fatigue is always there. Nothing is easy for either the stroke patient or the family caregiver. The caregiver finds themselves exhausted both physically and emotionally. It is a natural consequence of giving so much of oneself to the care of others. Those caregivers who are most dedicated to the profession are the ones most likely to experience burnout. The best thing to do is to recognize the symptoms and take steps to take care of yourself.

Family members and caregivers need to nurture themselves and take care of their own needs. The person that you are caring for needs you to be the best care provider you can be. You need to be physically healthy, alert, supportive, and loving. They depend on you, so you need to take good care of yourself so that you can take good care of them. As we all know, too much stress is bad for anyone and over time, can increase the risk of health problems. Too often, caregivers devote so much time to the health of their loved one, that they do not realize how their health and well-being is affected. The most effective, responsible, and healthy caregivers are those that attend to their individual emotional, physical, mental, and spiritual needs.

Here are the most common symptoms of caregiver stress or burnout that you should be aware of

- Fatigue.
- Frequent feelings of being overwhelmed.
- Constant worry.
- Changes in sleep patterns.
- Changes in weight and diet.
- Increased agitation.
- Bouts of anger.
- Depression.
- Loneliness.
- Frequent headaches.
- Abuse of alcohol, drugs, or prescription medications.
- Overreacting to minor nuisances.
- Trouble concentrating.
- Feeling resentful.
- Neglecting responsibilities.
- Impatience and irritability.
- Feeling helpless and hopeless.
-

There are activities in this book that would be beneficial for caregivers to use. They include journal writing, guided imagery sessions, and story-telling exercises. As well as music and art activities which are powerful stress busters.

RESPITE

Everyone needs a break from caregiving duties, even the most stoic of caregivers. Sometimes, a caregiver needs to hear from someone else that it is OKAY to take time out for themselves and not to feel guilty about it. It is vital that you give yourself some relief so that you are refreshed and energized to return to the demanding responsibilities of caring for another. Just imagine if you worked for a company for one or two years without ever taking a weekend or holiday off. How would that affect the quality of your life? It is important to understand that it is not only OKAY but vital that you take time for yourself.

I encourage you to set aside a minimum of an hour each day for yourself. During this time, you will not be doing anything for anyone but yourself. By scheduling time for this self-care, you are taking steps to restore some balance into your life. Find time to do the things you enjoy, whether it is working in the garden, exercising, reading, or keeping a journal. Stepping away to find time for yourself might feel like you are pampering yourself. There is nothing wrong with that; everyone needs a little pampering now and again. Pamper yourself with a massage, a long soak in the bathtub, a manicure, or even a nap. Do whatever makes you feel good. Be sure to get out of the house on your own during the week. Have lunch with friends or take a walk. If you cannot get out of the house, invite friends to visit. It is vital to maintain those connections to friends and family members. It allows you to share your feelings and receive feedback from those who care about you.

Too often, family caregivers neglect certain areas or activities in their life that were once important to them. They worry about leaving their loved one in another's care; they think they might be "abandoning" them." Instead of having those thoughts, consider instead that your loved one might enjoy the opportunity to meet new people or have a change of scenery. There are adult care centers and short-term nursing homes that are all possible respite solutions. AARP and the American Stroke Association, along with caregiver organizations, offer excellent tips. They have respite plans that can help you take the first step towards restoring balance in your life and reconnecting with yourself. I strongly encourage you to take time for those things that are important to your well-being.

SUPPORT GROUPS

I cannot stress enough the importance of finding a good support group. Members of support groups meet to discuss their experiences, share ideas, and provide emotional support for one another. A good support group is like gold, but if you cannot find one, and you can always start your own! One of the best things about support groups is realizing that you are not alone in the world. It is comforting to know that others have similar experiences. When you walk into a support group, it is like entering another world where strangers instantly connect from a single event--a stroke. A support group can offer suggestions and give new perspectives. There are also online stroke support groups that you can explore.

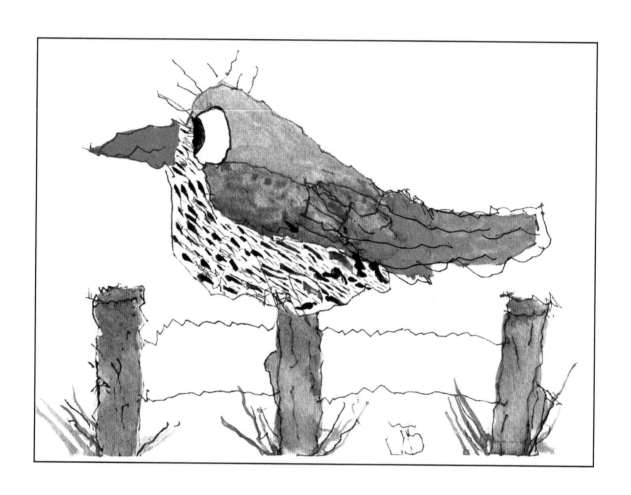

CHAPTER FOUR

COGNITIVE COACHING

A cognitive coach focuses on improving the thinking skills of their client and provides additional hours of focused cognitive training and activities. Coaches can be professional caregivers who, along with helping the patient with bathing, feeding, and other activities of daily living, also spend time doing cognitive work with the patient. A cognitive coach can also be an entirely different individual whose only responsibility is coaching.

Can a family member be a cognitive coach? Of course, they can, but they should remember that their most important role is being a family member! A wife or husband should not lose sight of the essence of their relationship: intimacy, laughter, sharing memories, having special moments, etc. Someone else can be the coach, but no one else can be a spouse. A husband or wife, who is the primary care provider, already has their hands full. They are running the household and taking care of their loved one's daily needs at the same time. Adding the role of cognitive coach is too much for one person to handle. However, they can add everyday experiences that stimulate cognition. Activities such as watching movies, and talking about them, playing games, going on outings together, are all great cognitive stimulators.

Let us assume for a moment that the primary family caregiver has decided to add a cognitive coach to the rehab team. How can they find someone suitable to perform this role? What are the attributes needed? What kind of background would be helpful?

TRAITS OF A GOOD COGNITIVE COACH

In my opinion, every coach or caregiver should possess the attributes on the list below. They also should be able to think critically and creatively and have strong interpersonal and communication skills. They will need to be able to organize activities, research information, do assessments, keep records, and follow instructions. The cognitive coach needs to be willing to form a relationship with the client built out of honesty, trust, and non-judgment.

Let us look at the "must-have" attributes of a cognitive coach or caregiver.

Alertness: Ability to observe when the client is struggling more than usual with the activity and be alert for signs of illness, depression, or sadness that come up.

Sensitivity: Ability to be sensitive to the ever-changing moods and physical and mental conditions of the client. Knowing how to select the right activity at the right moment under the right conditions and be willing to be flexible.

Patience: Rehabilitation coaching is not easy work, and it requires extreme patience to observe the painstakingly slow progress that it takes for their client to complete an exercise. A damaged brain that is busy repairing itself will naturally be slower to perform cognitive functions than a normal, healthy one. I have watched Jo take more than 30 minutes to complete an activity that usually would take a first grader less than 10 minutes. Her brain was undergoing tremendous work as it attempted to rebuild connections.

Creativity: An essential trait that a cognitive coach will use every day. Coaches will need to come up with creative activities and exercises. The ability to "think out of the box" is a valuable trait.

Compassionate: No one should be a cognitive coach or part of any rehabilitation team without this trait! A compassionate person is one that is aware of another's pain and suffering and feels a tenderness or empathy towards them.

Empathetic: The ability to put oneself in another's shoes and understand a person's emotions or feelings is empathy. If you do not take the time to understand what someone feels or is going through, then how can you fulfill their needs? It is a good reminder to ask yourself occasionally: What would it be like if I could not use my dominate hand? What would it be like if I could not speak or walk?

Honesty: Any person who works on the rehabilitation team needs to be honest and trustworthy. The primary care provider needs assurance that their loved one is with someone they can trust and gives them honest feedback. Most importantly, for progress to happen, the stroke client needs to be able to develop a relationship of trust with their coach.

Positivity: A cognitive coach will encounter challenges that can be very stressful and even disheartening while working with a client. A positive outlook is paramount. It will help

both the coach and client surmount the inevitable setbacks that the recovery path brings, including such as illness, depression, or frustration felt by the client.

COGNITIVE COACHES CAN COME FROM MANY BACKGROUNDS

Speech, physical therapy students, retired nurses, and professional caregivers would all make good cognitive coaches. Student teachers or retired teachers who know how to develop lesson plans that appeal to different learning styles would be excellent too. A retired teacher may love to put their skills back to use as a cognitive coach, or a student teacher might be anxious to put classroom theory into practice. Artists, musicians, movement specialists, and (dancers/massage therapists) have skills that could translate well into cognitive training.

There are essential factors to consider when looking for a cognitive coach. They need to know how to communicate information (teach) in a clear, understandable manner that is appropriate for the stroke patient. They should be able to evaluate performance accurately and make the necessary adaptations to the cognitive program.

RESPONSIBILITIES OF A COGNITIVE COACH

- Be able to create lesson plans or activities to support a specific objective that is realistic and measurable.

- Demonstrate knowledge or willingness to use other methods for communication (gestures, signs, images, electric devices).

- Be able to adapt activities to the changing needs and requirements of the client.

- Observe the client's progress and communicate information with family members or the primary care provider.

- Provide support (emotional, physical, and mental) to the client during sessions.

- Keep progress logs and reports accurately.

- Be aware of the client's limitations.

- Consider the client's safety and wellbeing above everything else.

- Maintain confidentiality.

PERSONALIZED COGNITIVE RECOVERY PROGRAM

A speech therapist or physical therapist may give the stroke survivor exercises to do at home. These exercises are "homework" and practiced between professional therapy visits. You can always be creative and add your ideas to this plan based on your client's additional needs and desires. Be sure to update the therapist with new additions whenever possible. Open communication between members on the recovery team makes all the difference in the world!

Client Information

The more you can understand about your client, the better chances you have of developing an effective, personalized cognitive plan. Find out as much information as you can from the primary caregiver or family member and client about the following:

- Client's age
- Personality characteristics
- Level of risk tolerance
- Interests and hobbies
- Work experience
- Educational level
- Significant relationships
- Level of exercise before the stroke event
- Motivators
- Joys, dreams, and goals

- Fears
- Likes and dislikes

Diagnosis

Questions to ask: What type of brain injury? What is the damage and to what extent? When did the damage occur? What is the prognosis for recovery?

Rehabilitation Team

Questions to ask: What professionals are part of the recovery team? How often are the sessions? What is occurring during these sessions? What are the goals and directives of the medical professionals?

Recovery Goals

What are the family's recovery goals for the client?
What are the client's goals?
What are the expectations for the cognitive coach?

Cognitive Sessions

How many cognitive recovery sessions per week? What is the length of the sessions? Will there be breaks scheduled for coach and client? Where will these sessions take place?

It is essential to have a clear understanding of the problems and levels of severity that your client is facing physically, emotionally, and cognitively. Without this information, you will be unable to create a plan that addresses specific goals and objectives. If possible, find out what cognitive abilities are compromised, (attention or problem-solving) the extent of damage, chances of recovery, and what can be done to improve it. Most professional treatment plans document six things: (1) Problems or limitations, (2) Levels of severity, (3) Analysis of underlying causes of difficulties, (4) Length of treatment, (5) Goals, and (6) Short-term objectives.

Once you have a plan, share it with the primary caregiver or family members and with the medical professionals of the rehab team. Ask for feedback, especially from the client. It is important to share the plan with the client because their understanding and acceptance of the treatment or recovery plan is a vital part of their progress. A survivor will feel more involved and motivated when they understand the "what, why, when and how" of their recovery plan.

The progress journal can be very simple or complex, depending on what you are comfortable doing. I write the date of the session and record Jo's physical condition, mood, pain level, and any comments that she made about her health at the beginning of the session. When we did motor exercises, my journals contained "logs," detailing the type of activity, the number of repetitions, and the amount of assistance that was needed. When we did language and cognitive exercises, I would record the length of time it took her to complete them. I would also note the number of cues required, and any other information that seemed significant.

I would also record Jo's comments as well and any concerns that came up during the session. The progress journal was handy for providing information to Dennis when he wanted to update the doctors. It is so easy to forget

KEEPING A PROGRESS JOURNAL

There are several reasons to keep a progress journal. It contains information about your client that you can reference when you communicate with family members. It is a chronological record of the client's progress. Within your progress journal, you might ask yourself questions such as:

1. What happened during the session?

2. Were goals and objectives met?

3. What exercises worked? What did not? Why?

4. What type of assistance or cues did the client need? How often?

5. How long did it take the client to complete a specific activity?

6. Was the client willing, cooperative, and able to perform tasks?

7. Was the client experiencing pain or illness?

8. What was the client's level of alertness?

9. Was there progress made, or did a setback occur from the previous session?

10. What problems are happening?

11. Were there activities that required adaptations?

12. What were the comments your client made about their progress?

13. Additional comments that you might want to add.

14. Date the entry.

what happens from day to day basis, but by jotting it down in a progress journal, it is always there for reference. I took the progress journal a step further and used it to compile quarterly "assessments" which I gave to her husband. I strongly encourage you to maintain a progress journal.

OBSERVE YOUR CLIENT

Jo's physical, emotional, and mental conditions changed almost every day. From our very first session, I felt it was essential to observe and record these changes in a journal. What did I look for when I sat down with Jo? I began each session, watching whether she seem tired, distracted, depressed, or energetic and alert. I observed her eyes to see if she could maintain contact with me or if her pupils were racing back and forth. I looked at how she was holding her body; was her posture reasonably straight, or was she slumped in her chair? Was she managing her secretions, or was she drooling significantly? Was her voice soft and breathy, or could I hear clear sounds?

Next, I would ask her if she was experiencing any discomfort or pain. If she had pain, I asked her to tell me or point to the pain area. We had established a pain monitoring scale from zero to 10, with zero being no pain and 10 being the worst pain. I would always explain the pain scale every time I asked her to describe the pain. It is a good idea to have this list typed up or to have a range of "frowning" faces to indicate the level of pain. Your client can point to the face or number to indicate their pain level. There are many examples online that you can download and print out. Here is the one I used:

0	No pain
1-2	Mild pain, but can do most activities
3-4	Moderate pain, but can, can do most activities with rest breaks
5-6	Uncomfortable pain, but can do limited activities with rest breaks
7	Extremely uncomfortable, restricted movement. Needs extended breaks.
8	Intense pain
9-10	Unbearable pain

ACTIVE AND EMPATHETIC LISTENING

Listening to your client is one of the best gifts you can give them. Every human being needs to feel that they are "heard" and to have their feelings or thoughts acknowledged without judgment. Helping someone who is having difficulty understanding and expressing their thoughts helps that person feel that they have something valuable to contribute to the conversation.

The best way to do this is to use active and empathic listening skills. Active listening is a technique where you repeat back to the person what you think she or he said to make sure you understand. You can say something like, "This is what I heard you say..." Ask clarifying questions to be sure that your client understands you. Let your client know that you want to understand them. Be patient and let the stroke survivor take as long as is needed, especially if they have aphasia. Empathetic listening involves putting yourself in someone else's position and trying to feel what it is that they are feeling. It includes paying attention to all verbal and nonverbal cues such as facial expressions, body language, and even tone of voice.

Often, what is not said speaks louder than what is said! The times when Jo would share her feelings with me, I would always acknowledge her feelings by saying, "It sounds like you are happy or worried about something." This acknowledgment allowed her to expand on her feelings or concerns. It is vital that when you are listening with empathy, that you give your total attention to that person, especially eye contact. When we finished talking, I would always thank her for sharing and let her know I would maintain confidentiality.

KEEP IT POSITIVE!

Those on the rehab team must maintain a hopeful and positive attitude when working with a stroke patient. Stroke survivors have not lost their sensitivity to their environment or to those that are in it. They may even be "hyper-sensitive" to everyone and everything around them. Often during the long, steep road of recovery, they may be prone to despair or a sense of hopelessness or helplessness. They will need a coach who is optimistic, joyful, and who will help encourage them through the challenges. If the coach believes in the ability of the client and shows it with a positive, upbeat attitude, it helps the client to believe in themselves.

Here is an example of two different coaching styles.

A Compassion Coach is the "cheerleader" who focuses on what the person CAN do at the moment and presents opportunities or learning experiences that expand on those abilities. Emphasis is on hope and positive outcomes. Past and current accomplishments, no matter how small, are recognized. The coach may use humor and light-heartedness to get their message across. The message usually given is, **You are good enough just as you are.**

A Compliance Coach is the "fixer," who focuses on the problem and emphasizes all the things that the person is doing wrong or what they cannot achieve. This type of coach is future-orientated and does not appreciate what is happening in the present moment. They continuously tell the individual that to accomplish something, they have to do it a certain way. The message given by this coach is, **You are not good enough until...**

Researchers at Case Western Reserve University have used brain images to see the effects of coaching with compassion versus coaching for compliance. Compassionate coaching produces something called the Positive Emotional Attractor (PEA). PEA produces positive emotions in the person coached. It arouses the neuroendocrine systems that stimulate better cognitive function and increased perceptual accuracy. Whereas the Negative Emotional Attractor (NEA), which emphases weaknesses, flaws, or other shortcomings, has the opposite effect.

"We're trying to activate the parts of the brain that would lead a person to consider possibilities," said Richard Boyatzis, distinguished university professor and professor of organizational behavior, cognitive science, and psychology. "We believe that would lead to more learning. By considering these possibilities, we facilitate learning. "If you focus on the negative, you will activate the Negative Emotional Attractor (NEA), which causes people to defend themselves, and as a result, they close down," Boyatzis says. [1]

I cannot stress enough how important it is that your interactions with your clients are positive, hopeful, inspirational, and motivating. There are many ways to do this. On those dark days, when Jo was feeling very hopeless, we would read inspirational passages, watch motivational videos, and talk about them. Other times, I would ask her to tell me about the times in her life when she faced and overcame challenges. Sometimes, just listening with empathy is the best thing to do.

IMPORTANT REMINDERS FOR COGNITIVE COACHES AND CAREGIVERS

- Use a normal conversational tone of voice to speak to your client.

- Be sure to look at your client when you are talking or explaining an activity.

- Position yourself at the same level as your client. Sit if the client is sitting.

- Avoid finishing your client's sentences.

- Give the client enough time to gather their thoughts and speak.

- Admit when you do not understand your client, but do so in a positive way.

- Have images and printed words available so the client can point to them.

- Always include your client in conversations with other people.

- Practice active and empathetic listening.

- Observe your client and record your observations.

- Monitor your client's pain level and make adaptations.

- Recognize when your client is feeling depressed and find ways to change their attitude.

- Identify and maximize your client's strengths.

ALWAYS BEGIN EACH SESSION WITH A POSITIVE ATTITUDE

AND END EACH SESSION ON A POSITIVE NOTE!

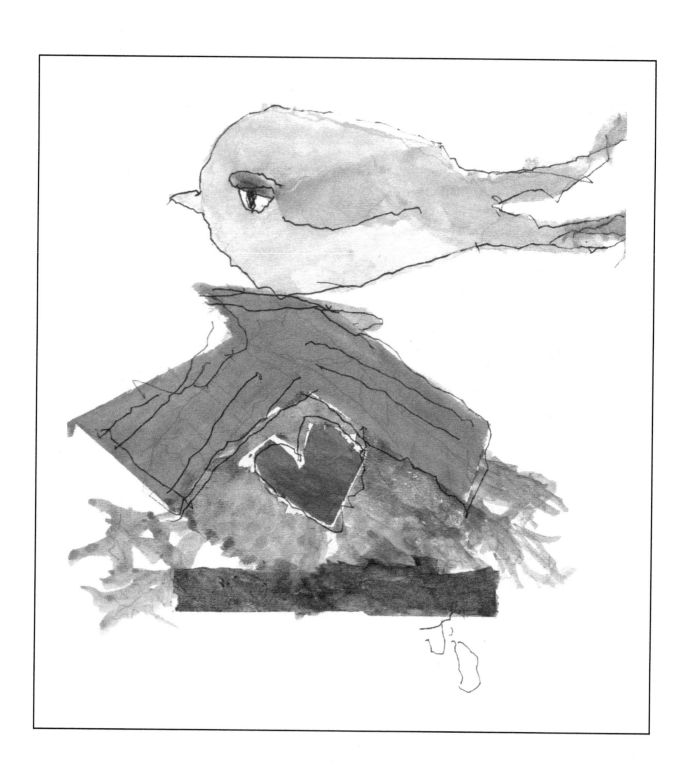

CHAPTER FIVE

GOALS AND OBJECTIVES

True teachers are those who use themselves as bridges over which they invite their students to cross; then, having facilitated their crossing, joyfully collapse, encouraging them to create their own. —Nikos Kazantzakis

There is a strong consensus among rehabilitation experts that the most critical elements in any rehabilitation program are well-focused goals and objectives, along with repetitive practice. Goals will be patient-specific, but here is a list of goals that are common for stroke survivors:

- Improve mobility.
- Improve balance
- Increase strength.
- Increase range of motion.
- Increase endurance.
- Improve fine motor skills.
- Improve cognition - memory, learning, and awareness.
- Improve speech.
- Understand spoken and written language.
- Improve swallowing.
- Reduce pain.
- Improve vision.

- Reduce negative emotions: depression, lack of motivation, fear, hopelessness, etc.
- Complete activities of daily living (toiletry, eating, dressing, etc.) independently.
- Return to driving.
- Return to work.
- Return to independence.

HOW TO SET GOALS

If you want to achieve something, you have to know what it is you want to achieve. So, how does one go about knowing what they what to achieve? As a coach, how do you help your client achieve their recovery goals? First step is to have a concrete GOAL. Goals are usually general in scope. Examples of general goals would be "improve mobility" or "increase memory." Goals are the big picture. One of the methods I used to establish goals and leaning objectives in this program was S.M.A.R.T., the acronym commonly attributed to Peter Drucker. [1]

SMART goals are:

Specific	(simple, sensible, significant).
Measurable	(meaningful, motivating).
Achievable	(agreed, attainable).
Relevant	(reasonable, realistic and resourced, results-based).
Time bound	(time/cost limited, time-sensitive).

Specific goals focus on answering the following questions:

- What do you want to accomplish?
- What do you want your client to know?
- What do you want your client to do?
- Why is this goal important?
- Where will this take place?
- How will it take place?
- When will it take place?

Measurable goals focus on answering the following question:

- How will you know when it is accomplished?

Achievable goals focus on answering the following questions:

- Is it realistic?
- Is it achievable?
- Is there time available?
- Are there resources available?
- What limitations are involved?

Relevant goals answer the following questions:

- Is it worthwhile?
- Is this the right time for this goal?
- Is it appropriate for the situation, circumstance or individual?

Time-bound goals answer the following questions:

- How long will it take to accomplish this goal?
- What can be done on a daily basis?
- What can be done on a weekly or monthly basis?
- What is the goal for six months from now, or a year from now?

HOW TO DETERMINE OBJECTIVES

Now that you have some idea about establishing goals, you will need to know how to narrow down those goals into clear objectives.

1. Select the rehabilitation goal.
2. Determine the specific, focused objectives needed to support each desired goal.
3. Determine the activities or actions (steps) needed to achieve the objective.
4. Determine the criteria that used to assess success.
5. Evaluate effectiveness of activities and actions to meet objective and make appropriate changes.

Let us look at two of the broad goals from the above list of rehabilitation goals: "increase mobility" and "improve cognitive skills." Both goals are very broad-based and on their own may seem to be a massive undertaking. That is why it is important to establish objectives for each goal. Objectives take the broad goal and break it down into understandable, measurable steps. Having a clear objective will help you design activities that are relevant and provide a basis for assessment. Let us say we decide the first objective for achieving the above goal will be to focus on improving balance. With this clear objective in mind, we can consider ways to accomplish it through action steps.

Goal: Increase Mobility
Objective: Improve Balance
Motor Skill Activity: Standing

Action Steps:

1. Perform sit to stand exercises: 10 repetition, 3 times daily.

2. Stand at counter: 5 minutes, three times daily.

3. Holding onto chair, bend one leg at the knee and hold for 5 seconds.

Evaluation:

1. How were the action steps accomplished? (How many repetitions achieved? How many times?)

2. How did the client perform (legs shaky or body tilted)?

3. Did the client feel pain, dizziness, fear, excitement or confusion? Are adjustments in repetitions or adaptable equipment needed?

Goal: Improve Cognitive Skills
Objective: Improve Memory
Activity: Reading

Action Steps:

1. Listen or read a story aloud.

2. Remember the main points of the story.

3. Client retells the story in their own words.

Evaluation:

1. Was the client able to follow along with story?

2. Did the client have trouble concentrating?

3. Was the client able to remember the main points of the story?

4. Did the client have trouble using language skills to answer the questions?

5. How long did it take the client to answer these questions?

6. Are there any adjustments needed? (Large letters, more time to respond, cues, etc.)

To recap,

1. Define the rehabilitation goal.

2. Determine specific objectives to support that goal.

3. Define actions steps to accomplish the objective.

4. Understand how to evaluate progress.

SUGGESTIONS FOR EFFECTIVE ACTIVITIES AND EXERCISES

In the early stages of cognitive recovery, I would suggest that the client be provided brilliant images in the form of movies or picture books or photographs. Provide them opportunities to hear a variety of pleasant music and stories on tape. When possible organize as many new experiences or sensations as can be tolerated. As your client improves, their brain will require more challenges. As a cognitive coach, you will want to be sensitive for when these shifts occur. Present exercises and activities that they are within reach of your client, yet not too easy and not too hard. Easy activities may bring temporary satisfaction but little challenge. While exercises that are too challenging can cause feelings of frustration or hopelessness.

It was a trial and error process to determine activities and exercises to use with Jo. Some things worked, somethings did not. Keep in mind that an activity or exercise that is too difficult initially, might be easier to handle a few weeks or months later. In addition, during the recovery period and beyond, certain conditions might interfere with leaning. These conditions could be physical: vision difficulties, limited movement, tiredness, pain, low concentration and illness. There could be emotional issues such as depression or fear that surface when working with your client. It is important to be able to observe what works and what does not and make changes accordingly. Experiment and evaluate!

Dr. Benjamin Bloom's Taxonomy, created in 1956, focuses on promoting higher forms of thinking in education, such as analyzing and evaluating concepts, processes, procedures, and principles, rather than just remembering facts (rote learning). The taxonomy is useful when designing educational, training, and learning processes. I used this taxonomy as well as the S.M.A.R.T. goals when selecting activities for Jo.

Cognitive Learning Objective:

1. What do I want Jo to know?

2. What do I want Jo to do?

3. do I want Jo to feel?

Level of Challenge:

1. Is this activity considered: easy, moderate or hard?

2. Is the level of challenge equal to the client's cognitive and motor abilities?

3. Does this activity encourage new learning?

4. Does this exercise require the client to draw from past memory, knowledge or experience to do this activity?

Level of Effectiveness:

1. Was the learning objective accomplished?

2. Was the activity completed in a reasonable length of time?

3. How well was the client able to perform activity?

4. Was client able to adjust to the pace and timing of the activity?

5. How well was the information processed or understood?

6. Were there many requests for repeated information or directions?

After each lesson, I asked myself how much assistance I was providing as a coach. How often was physical assistance or visual and verbal cues provided? Was I giving more aid than the exercise should have required, indicating that perhaps it was too difficult for the client at this stage? Did the exercise appear too easy? You can use the same exercise over again and as often as it is needed and desirable, just as long as you continue to add new challenges to it. I believe the best way to increase challenge is in incremental, obtainable steps rather than attempting to leap over huge hurdles.

Assessments show measurable gains or progress over time. It is an opportunity to re-evaluate activities and see if they are effective (evidenced by cognitive or motor progress) and if appropriate, to make changes. This requires objectivity, good observational and record keeping skills. Your assessments should show how you measured progress over several weeks or months. First, decide how often you will do your assessments, there is no hard and fast rule for this. I would suggest after your first month, you go through your progress notes and complete your first assessment. As you reflect on the assessment, you will be able to draw conclusions about the exercises and activities you presented and make any needed adaptations.

PATIENT-CENTERED GOALS

Patient-centered goals involves the active participation and contribution of the patient to their own recovery. These goals trigger motivation, self-responsibility, self-initiation and self-awareness. It is important to talk about the rehabilitation goals with the stroke survivor and discuss ways they can accomplish the goals. Ask them what type of assistance and adaptations they would like. Encourage them to have active participation in this process. This is the "buy in" moment!

These steps are important in the patient-centered goal process:

1. Patient and coach have a clear understanding of the goals.

2. Coach provides cues, aids or physical assistance as needed.

3. Patient attempts to complete the task and meet the focused goal.

4. Coach observes patient as they attempt task.

5. After an activity is completed, patient is encouraged to spend a few moments reflecting on the outcome of the activity.

6. Coach can encourage feedback by asking:

> Do you feel you were successful in completing the task?
> What went well?
> What was the most difficult?
> What could be improved?

Coach and patient should discuss any necessary changes needed to achieve the objective next time. Patient centered goals promote feelings of self-satisfaction and accomplishment, which only leads to a greater desire to accomplish more. I believe that desire and motivation are critical both in cognitive and physical rehabilitation. The moment I realized this was true was when I saw Jo, wiggling and stretching her body forward to accomplish an art and music activity. She was initiating these movements herself because it was something she really wanted to do!

HOW TO MEASURE PROGRESS

When you are recording your session notes, consider the following questions. They will help you gauge how well and how quickly your client is progressing.

GENERAL ASSESSMENT QUESTIONS

1. Were the directions and target goal clearly understood?

2. How much assistance was provided, such as cueing or physical assistance?

3. How many requests for repeat information?

4. How long was the client able to maintain attention on the task?

5. Did the client's physical limitations, if any, affect or interfere with the performance of this activity?

6. How long did the exercise or activity take?

7. Was the client able to articulate their experience about this activity?

The following is a compilation from the research I did regarding the brain and its cognition functions. This information was one of the most valuable things I learned from studying the brain and cognition. It helped me create activities to exercise each thinking skill as well as to target several skills at once. It helped me understand that our brains think in many ways.

1. **Attention:** Ability to stay focused.

2. **Comprehension:** Ability to understand new information and recall that information.

3. **Memory:** Ability to remember recent moments and past memories.

4. **Association:** Ability to know how two things are the same and how they are different.

5. **Processing:** Speed the brain processes both auditory and visual information.

6. **Sequencing:** Understanding the stages from large to small.

7. **Cognitive Flexibility:** Ability to shift thinking and attention between different things.

8. **Categorizing:** Ability to sort objects with other similar objects.

9. **Decision-making:** Ability to sort through information and make logical decisions.

10. **Flexibility:** Ability to switch to different thinking modes.

11. **Emotional Self-Regulation:** Ability to manage emotions.

12. **Task Shifting:** Ability to shift attention between one task and another. Ability to do more than one task at a time.

13. **Pattern Recognition**: Ability to see patterns in things.

14. **Perception**: Ability to see, hear or become aware of something through the senses.

15. **Language:** Ability to communicate thoughts and feelings appropriately.

16. **Motivation**: Ability to initiate an activity or movement.

17. **Problem Solving:** Ability to solve a specific problem with using critical and creative thinking processes.

18. **Reasoning:** Ability to think in a manner that leads to conclusions or judgments. Includes: deductive and inductive.

19. **Abstract Thinking:** Ability to process complex ideas that usually not concrete or visible.

20. **Analyzing:** Ability to examine something in close detail and make determinations.

21. **Creativity:** Ability to use the imagination and imagery to come up with new ideas, things or solutions.

22. **Monitoring performance:** Ability to observe one's own performance.

23. **Fine Motor Skills:** Ability to coordinate eye and hand movements along with control hand and finger movements.

PART II

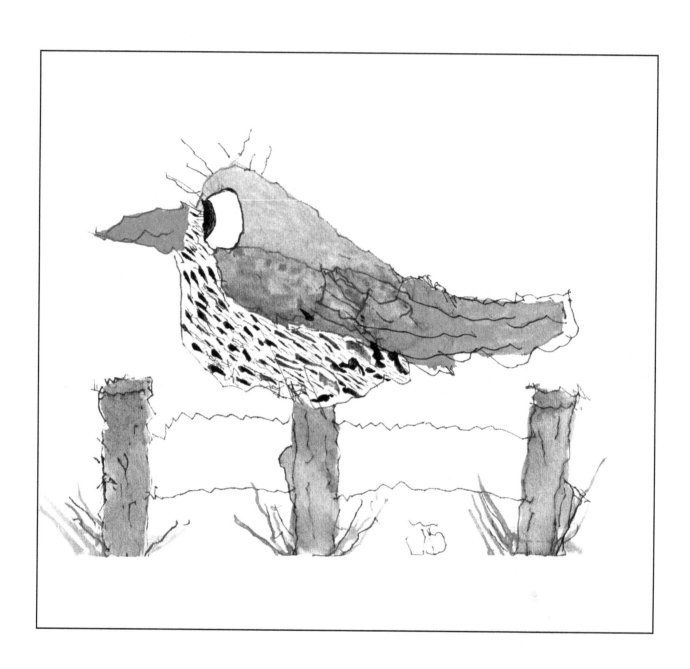

CHAPTER SIX

COMMUNICATION AFTER STROKE

The limits of my language means the limits of my world. —Ludwig Wittgenstein

Regaining speech skills after stroke is similar to learning a new language for the first time. It is not easy. Jo had a tracheotomy tube in her throat for a little over a year and a half, and her vocal cords were not functioning correctly. This certainly made it very difficult for her to control her secretions, clear her throat, swallow, and manage her breath. It was only after her tracheotomy tube was removed, and after vocal cord surgery, that her speech began to show improvement. After months of practice, Jo was finally able to produce audible sounds versus breathy sounds. However, the fluency of her speech and her articulation and volume were poor. Swallowing continued to challenge Jo even with constant reminders. She usually had to make several attempts at a cleansing swallow to remove all her secretions. Later, I found that when we were singing, she did a better job clearing her throat, maybe because her vocal cords vibrated more from singing.

Jo's facial and jaw muscles were extremely tight, and she would often complain that she felt pain in her jaw. I began our speech sessions with a short facial massage to help loosen the jaw and cheek muscles. Each day we worked on the vowel sounds (A, E, I, O, U). We stretched our facial muscles by exaggerating the movement it took to make those sounds. Other exercises we did focused on practicing difficult sounds. Several sounds require clear diction to be distinguished from each other. An example would be the sounds: "T," "D," and "B" and "P" and words like "chin and skin," or "chop and shop." Sometimes we used a device (voice wave) that amplified her sounds so she could hear them. This helped her to realize how she sounded instead of what she thought she said. Instead of this device, a simple voice recorder would be helpful. As Jo's speech improved, I added exercises on language, association, categorizing, naming, alphabetizing, spelling, and reading, which kept things varied for her.

Practicing speech can be challenging and exhausting for a stroke survivor, so be sure to take frequent breaks. It is good to find ways to be creative with the voice and sounding exercises since the drills can become boring. One thing that was fun to do was to sing silly songs and recite tongue twisters! There is not anything that you can do wrong in the practicing of speech, except by allowing poor diction. A lazy tongue will only lead to lazy speech. Just like a fitness coach in a gym, you want to encourage your client to do one more "tongue push" or pronounce another word. Drills can be tedious, but they are necessary to improve speech. Repetition is the key to accomplishing this goal.

For the first five- or six-years post stroke, Jo's communication skills slowly improved, although she continued to have difficulty retrieving names for people and things. When I began working with Jo, she called everything "yellow." It must have been one of her favorite colors. Over time, she remembered more and more words as we practiced our vocabulary exercises. As Jo showed ability and interest, our language exercises advanced to writing and storytelling exercises which worked on her cognitive skills. The following is a wonderful example of Jo's ability to choose words and put them together to form a poem. Particularly impressive was her using the words "vision" and "roost," words not usually used in her daily conversation.

I fly with vision before me
I go below to get food and bring it to my children.
I get food for birds who can't gather it for themselves.
I tell other birds where they can find food.

I have wings and I can fly high up in the sky.
I also have an area to roost upon.
It has flowers and space to bring friends.
I bring food to birds that need it.
I show how to bring food to friends who need it.

The following clearly illustrates the hardship stroke survivors experience trying to regain their communication skills. Jo describes her condition very clearly and honestly

My voice is too quiet. And, it is too soft. And, it is too difficult for me to talk. Sometimes, people have difficulty in hearing me. I speak too quiet. And, I can't make myself talk loudly. I have to talk out of my mouth; I have to pronounce. I run out of energy when speaking loudly. The energy comes from my mouth and throat. I think the energy is a little bit more on the left side, but I am not sure.
I don't sound very loud to myself. It

doesn't ever sound very loud. When I try to make sounds, it is very difficult and most of the time it comes out confusing. It is difficult to talk all the time. I try to talk louder for people to understand me but I don't really end up talking loudly. It is always a problem to talk more loudly. I don't know why. I always run out of breath. I don't want to talk or say anything unless it's necessary, because my voice sounds too little. No one can understand me. I cannot speak clearly. I have to try to talk loudly. It's tiring. My mouth gets tired. It feels stiff.

I feel like I am left out. Nobody wants to talk to me. I don't know what to say. I don't want to sound stupid. I don't know what to do or what to try. They don't understand how I feel. I can't talk with them. They don't know what I am saying so they make up words that they think I mean. I just say ok when this happens. It answers their questions. I feel badly that I can't talk. I need more time to talk. When the conversation is fast or a lot of people are talking, I can't be included. I don't have the time I need to talk. I feel I need more time then they use. What I miss about having a conversation is feeling closer to people.

TIPS FOR COMMUNICATING WITH A STROKE SURVIVOR

1. Speak Slowly.

It is especially important to remember that stroke survivors need extra time to formulate their thoughts and to choose their words. There is a lot of activity going on in their minds as they process the auditory statement or question and then find the words they wish to use. When I asked Jo what she needed me to do when communicating, she suggested that I speak slowly and allow her extra time to respond. She also mentioned that multiple conversations and loud background noise caused her to become distracted or confused when she tried to think.

2. Give Extra Time For A Verbal Response.

Whenever I asked Jo a question it would take her several moments to respond. I would ask her if she understood what I asked or what I just said. If she said no, I would rephrase the question. Sometimes, I would ask her to repeat what she thought I said. Often, she would relay the information correctly, using words of her choosing.

It was very important for me to reward Jo for her efforts every time she communicated. I wanted her to know that she was a person who had something to say and was worth listening to. This positive feedback encouraged her to talk and take the risk of making a mistake. Sometimes, I would smile and tell her, "That's an interesting response," which usually made us both giggle.

3. Be Encouraging.

Establishing a safe, non-judgmental communication environment is very important in helping stroke survivors practice their language skills. It was important because Jo had developed doubts about her ability to communicate. By removing any pressure to speak quickly, she could relax and let her thoughts flow more easily.

I also noticed that when she felt insecure in coming up with an answer or response, her voice would lower, and her words became muffled and difficult to understand. It happened often enough to make me realize one of two things might be happening: 1) All her concentration was on finding the right word and not the proper mechanics of speaking, or 2) She was feeling insecure and lowered her voice so she would not be embarrassed.

Since I did not know what was causing this,

I chose to focus on the importance of pushing past her "I don't know" or "I can't remember" statements. I would repeat the parts of her sentences that I could understand leaving the gaps, alerting her to the words that were missing or misunderstood. I would repeat again, "This is what I heard you say." Is this correct?" This type of communication technique serves two purposes. It tells the stroke survivor that you sincerely want to understand and communicate with them and that you have the patience to wait for their response. Secondly, the stroke survivor can hear their words echoed back to them and maybe recognize the words they are having difficulty expressing.

Another useful technique is to have the stroke survivor speak into a tape recorder and let them hear their voice. Jo was amazed at how she sounded on tape. She had thought she was talking clearer and louder than she really was.

4. Keep Distractions To A Minimum.

Most of us can focus better if we do not have distractions competing for our attention. This is especially true for a stroke survivor who may still be struggling with language and concentration skills. Turn down the TV or music player when talking. Give them the best chance for success by eliminating auditory and visual distractions.

5. Try Rephrasing Statements or Questions

It is frustrating to keep repeating the same question to someone who does not understand it in the first place. Nothing gets accomplished and everyone ends up exasperated. Select simple, straightforward words and keep sentences short. Try rephrasing sentences and questions for clearer understanding.

6. Don't Correct Every Word Every Time

Encourage all attempts to communicate! It is best not to point out every word the stroke survivor speaks incorrectly. It will only contribute to frustration and lack of confidence. No one likes to have his or her mistakes pointed out continually. Instead, celebrate the successes, no matter how small. Focus on what is going well, not what is going wrong.

7. Give Cues As Needed

There are many ways to give a cue. If a cue is wanted, then begin by demonstrating the beginning sounds of the word. Say something like, "the word sounds like "bab," demonstrating the beginning sounds of the word "baby."

- Sometimes, you need to say more than the beginning sound. You might need to add syllables of the word, such as "cal" or "ca-len," for the word "cal-en-dar."

- Another cue is to give the opposite (ant-onym) of the word. Say, "The word you are looking for is the opposite of hot." You can suggest the synonym by saying, "The word you are looking for means the same as *tiny*." Rhyming may be a useful cue at times. Say, "The word you are looking for (sing) rhymes with "ring."

- If possible, show an image of the word you want your client to say.

- You can use common phrases that will stimulate their memory and help them say the word. If you want your client to say the word "bacon," you can say the phrase, "Eggs and ____" Jo did very well with common phrases. A list of common phrases is included later in this chapter.

- A statement using multiple cues might sound like this, "The word I am looking for begins with the letter 'C' and sounds like 'co' and means frigid or chilly (cold). What word do you think it is?"

- Another helpful cue is to provide multiple-choice answers for your client. Say, "Is the word, tree, candle, or cake?"

8. Ask The Stroke Patient What They Need.

Do not forget that the stroke patient needs to be involved whenever possible in decisions about their needs and rehabilitation. Do not assume something or attempt a technique without asking for their input. Their awareness may be quite surprising. Most of these tips were expressed to me by Jo when I asked her what needs to be done to help her communicate better and to help others understand her better.

WHAT TO EXPECT FROM THE SPEECH THERAPIST

Many stroke survivors experience a variety of communication challenges. The following list are some of the most common difficulties; although, it is not inclusive. Only a professional speech and language pathologist (SLP) can make a proper diagnosis. During the initial consultation, the speech therapist will assess the patient's ability to swallow and communicate. This includes testing for verbal comprehension as well as the patient's ability to express their thoughts in words.

Here are some of the major areas the SLP will focus on:

Swallowing: which can put the survivor at risk for complications like choking, coughing and even infection, as well as affect their enjoyment of eating. If your speech therapist diagnoses a swallowing problem, they will recommend specific exercises to strengthen the muscles used in swallowing and speech production. They can also recommend certain foods that are easier to swallow.

Difficulty in breathing: is a common problem for stroke patients. It contributes to their difficulty in completing sentences or phrases. Often, they have to draw a breath before they can finish a sentence.

Articulation: is the production of speech sounds generated by the proper placement and control of the speech muscles such as lips, teeth, jaw, soft palate and tongue for clarity in speech. The ability to imitate sound is also a measure of articulation.

Resonance: Resonance is the quality of voice that results from the sound vibrations in the oral, nasal and pharyngeal cavities during speech. Abnormal obstruction in these areas will affect the quality of speech.

Fluency: Fluency refers to the flow of speech. Dysfluency consists of pauses, prolonged sounds, or repetition of sounds and words.

Speech therapists will also test for cognitive ability by asking simple yes or no question. They will ask the patient to identify the proper sequence of activities. Which goes on first, shoes or socks? Which day of the week comes first, Monday or Wednesday? Other testing might include the patient's ability to recognize patterns, sort, categorize, make associations, and recall information. They will evaluate the cognitive skills of attention, memory, decision-making, reasoning, comparison, identifying, classification, and others.

Most stroke survivors meet with the speech therapist one to three times a week for about one hour. Frequency may vary depending on the needs of the patient, where they are in the rehabilitation process, and their insurance limitations.

Often the speech therapist will encourage family members to work on speech exercises at home to compliment the therapy sessions and to facilitate the speed of recovery. The next section will focus on some at-home exercises that will provide good practice in language skills.

SPEECH AND COMMUNICATION EXERCISES

I am not a medical professional and I do not intend to replace the work of a professional speech therapist, only to support it. The knowledge and experience that a speech therapist brings to the rehabilitation effort is very vital. Be sure that you check with them before beginning any of the following exercises. These professionals in the field will know what will work best for the stroke patient and what will not. The therapists will welcome your willingness to do "homework" and will probably suggest some exercises after the first session.

In designing this part of the program, I used the exercises that the speech therapist initially gave me, along with new ones from a variety of resources. Initially, the speech and communication goals set for Jo by the speech therapist were:

- Hold head upright.

- Increase swallowing frequency and control secretions.

- Improve strength and control of tongue.

- Loosen facial and jaw muscles.

- Articulate individual sounds distinctly.

- Control breathe while speaking.

- Improve memory.

- Improve ability to follow directions.

Most likely, your loved one or client will have some, if not all, of these goals to accomplish too. Ask the speech therapist what their specific goals are for the stroke patient. It is important to understand the goals to find ways to accomplish them. A typical session with a professional speech therapist lasts for about an hour. There is a good reason for this as the patient has limited energy and mental endurance. There is a point when no more new information can be taken in. It is important that as a coach, you are sensitive to this. My sessions with Jo were broken up into three areas: speech, motor skills and cognition. Since, our focus on this chapter is on speech and communication, here is a suggested schedule. Feel free to adjust according to your client's and your needs. Nothing about recovery is set in stone, especially schedules!

Use the first schedule for a stroke survivor who needs assistance regaining control of their speech muscles, voicing and articulation skills. It is a 60-minute session. You can supplement the session with 30 minutes of language skill and reading practice for a 90-minute session. The professional speech therapist should look over this schedule and add their own exercises or suggestions. For instance, the speech therapist may feel there is a need to devote more time to facial and oral motor exercises and less on language skills or vice versa.

SAMPLE SCHEDULE ONE

Facial massage	5 minutes
Breathing	5 minutes
Facial and Oral Motor Exercises	20 minutes
Articulation Exercises	15 minutes
Language Exercises	15 minutes
Total	**60 minutes**

SAMPLE SCHEDULE TWO

Facial Massage	5 minutes
Facial and Oral Motor Exercises	15 minutes
Articulation Exercises	20 minutes
Language Skills Exercises	30 minutes
Reading Exercises	20 minutes
Total	**90 minutes**

Remember, these schedules are just suggestions to help you get started. As you work with the stroke patient, you will find that some activities take longer or that the client's needs and abilities are changing each day. Just relax and go with the flow. Being there to help your client communicate is the most important thing; even if that means you just have a conversation with your client. Learning how to regain conversational skills is important. Every chance you can engage your stroke client in conversational speech is a "win" moment. So, on those tough days, when cognition ability seems lower than usual, talk about what is going on in your client's life, upcoming holidays, family events or current events. Just have fun talking together.

FACIAL AND ORAL MOTOR EXERCISES

1. Face Massage (10-15 minutes)

- Massage areas of face.

- Manual stretch – place right thumb inside left cheek and push outward firmly but gently.

- Place left thumb inside right cheek and push outward firmly but gently.

2. Facial Stretching Exercises:

- Raise your eyebrows as high as possible, then relax.

- Frown as hard as possible, wrinkle nose, and bring eyebrows together.

- Open your mouth as wide as you can, and stretch it as much as possible.

- Puff out your cheeks and stretch them as much as possible.

- Make exaggerated vowel sounds (A, E, I, O, U) stretching as much as possible.

- Move your jaw to the right side as far as you can until it pulls but does not hurt. Hold five seconds. Repeat five to ten times.

- Move your jaw to the left side as far as possible. Hold five seconds. Repeat five to ten times.

- Move your jaw around in a circle making it move as far in each direction as you can until you feel a stretch, but no pain. Repeat five times.

3. Lip Exercises

- Lip Retraction: Spread lips into a smile. Hold for five seconds. Relax and repeat ten times.

- Lip Protrusion: Pucker your lips as if you are going to give someone a kiss. Hold for five seconds. Relax and repeat ten times.

- Lip Retraction and Protrusion: Alternately smile and then pucker your lips. Use exaggerated movements. Relax and repeat ten times.

- Lip Press: Open mouth as wide as possible and hold for five seconds. Then close mouth. Press lips tightly together for five seconds. Relax and repeat ten times.

- Lip Press on Tongue Depressor: Tightly press lips around tongue depressor, while coach/caregiver tries to remove it. Perform for three to five seconds. Relax and repeat five times.

- Suck your lips into your mouth, then release in a loud smacking noise. Repeat ten times.

4. Tongue Exercises

Tongue tension can make the voice weak and cause it to sound nasally or mumbled.

- Open your mouth and protrude your tongue. Be sure your tongue is straight out, not resting on your lips or pointing to one side. Maintain this position for five to ten seconds. Do ten repetitions.

- Protrude your tongue and move it slowly from corner to corner over your lips. Do ten repetitions.

- Protrude tongue and point it upward toward nose, hold for five seconds, then relax. Do ten repetitions.

- Protrude tongue and point downward toward the chin, hold for five seconds. Do ten repetitions.

- Tongue Push Forward: Stick out your tongue as far as you can. Put tongue depressor or spoon against your tongue. Push against your tongue with the flat object at the same time you push against the flat object with your tongue. Hold for five seconds. Repeat five to ten times.

- Tongue Push Up: Push down on your tongue with the flat object, while at the same time you push up with your tongue. Hold for five seconds. Repeat five to ten times.

- Tongue inside Push: Put your finger against your right check about 1 inch to the side of the corner of your mouth. From the inside, push your tongue against your cheek where your finger is touching. Push as hard as you can. Hold for five seconds. Relax and repeat five times for each side of the mouth.

- Move tongue around your lips in a circle, touching all of upper lip, corners and lower lip. Practice ten times.

BREATHING EXERCISES

When we breathe correctly, we fill our lungs with air that circulates throughout our bodies providing nutrient to every cell. Every time we exhale deeply, we are ridding our body of carbon dioxide and toxins. When we take shallow breaths, our lungs are not fully exercised. This can have undesirable effects on our bodies. The following is a list of benefits that can happen with increased levels of oxygen in our bodies:

1. Improved digestion.
2. Lowered blood pressure and heart rate.
3. Reduced levels of stress hormones.
4. Improved immune system.
5. Increased physical energy.
6. Reduced lactic acid build-up in muscle tissue.
7. Increased nourishment for the nervous system improving health of the entire body.
8. Rejuvenation of the pituitary and pineal glands.
9. Rejuvenation of the skin.
10. Upper movement of the diaphragm massages the heart and stimulates blood circulation.
11. Deep breathing massages the abdominal organs, stomach, intestines, liver and pancreas.
12. Lungs become healthier and more efficient.
13. Relaxation of the mind and body, and reduction in anxiety.

Light-headedness or dizziness can occur with some of these exercises. If that happens, rest between repetitions or reduce repetitions and check with a medical professional. Usually, these symptoms will disappear after continued practice. Jo and I practiced breathing exercises before starting our vocal exercises for speech improvement. I found that it helped her become centered, focused and relaxed. It also brought her attention back to her body through the intimate process of breathing. Typically, we started with a deep cleansing breath (in through nose and out through mouth) to empty the lungs. Then we did the following breathing exercises:

Deep Breathe and Hold

1. Begin by sitting straight in a chair and taking a deep breath and expelling all air.

2. Inhale through the nose for a count of four, filling lungs as much as possible.

3. Hold breath for four counts.

4. Exhale completely through the mouth with a whooshing sound and pursed lips for a count of four.

5. Repeat five times.

We did a variation on this exercise by exhaling with clenched teeth while making the "ssss" sound. This was an excellent exercise for her because it helped her control the volume of air she was exhaling. I was hoping it would also help Jo manage her airflow as she spoke. This exercise induces a state of calm relaxation.

Huffing Breath

This technique will push air out of the lungs and can loosen mucus which can encourage coughing.

1. Take a normal breath in and out.

2. Take a normal breath in and force the air out of your mouth with a "huffing" sound. Your stomach muscles will contract.

3. Keep huffing out until no more air comes out.

4. Repeat 1-2 huffs then pause.

5. Do some deep breaths between huffing

6. Repeat two more times.

Diaphragmatic breathing

1. Begin by relaxing shoulders. Place one hand on your chest and the other on your belly.

2. Inhale through your nose for about two seconds.

3. As you breathe in, your belly should move outward. Your belly should move more than your chest.

4. As you breathe out slowly through pursed-lips, gently press on your belly. This will push up on your diaphragm and help get your air out.

Repeat four times.

The following activities are good for practicing pursing the lips as well as sustaining breath force and control:

Blowing through a straw to move a lightweight object (crumpled paper, feather, and cotton ball).
Blowing on a pinwheel.

Blowing soap bubbles.

Blowing a pencil across a flat surface. This requires stronger breath.

Blowing on a harmonica. Practice making loud and soft sounds and one note at a time.

Using a spirometer.

Horn blowing.

Blowing up balloons.

Whistling.

VOICING EXERCISES

ACTIVITY: Vocal Scales

This activity can assist with understanding pitch and stretching the vocal cords by singing the scales. Start from the low "Doh" note and slowly work your way up to the higher ranges. For a variation, try "Doh, Mi, Soi, Mi, Doh." Use a piano for this exercise if you can.

ACTIVITY: Humming

Practice humming to familiar songs. Humming helps with breath control, rhythm, memory and articulation.

ACTIVITY: Mm-mmm

Say "mm-mmm (sound you would say if something were yummy) Repeat 10 times.

Then alternate with the sound of "mmm-hmm" (sound you would say if you meant yes.) Repeat 10 times. Be sure your client's sounds are clear and distinguishable. Do not rush through this exercise; the goal is to make clear sounds. Your client should be able to feel some vibrations.

After this exercise is satisfactorily completed, then add another level of difficulty. Have your client go up and down their vocal range from low to high and back again using both sounds. Repeat 10 times.

ACTIVITY: Siren Sound

Make a siren sound using the sounds of "ooooo and eeeeee," traveling up and down the vocal scale. Try to get progressively higher with each attempt.

ACTIVITY: Lip Trill

The goal of this exercise is to vibrate the lips in a relaxed manner while making the "brrrr" sound and controlling breath. The sound is similar to a boat engine revving up in the water. If this is difficult to do at first, place one finger from each hand on each side of your face (where dimples would usually be). Do the exercise ten times. Then remove fingers and attempt to do the lip trill again. This is an excellent exercise to relax the lips.

ACTIVITY: Vocal Cord Adduction

1. Say "ah" while pushing down on chair. Repeat 10 times. Repeat sound while lifting up on chair.

2. Turn head to damaged side and say "ah." Repeat 10 times.

ACTIVITY: KA & TA Sounds

1. Say "ka" six times as clearly as possible. Repeat 10 times. To make this sound correctly, the throat needs to be clear and dry. The sound originates in the back of the throat.

2. Say "ta" six times as clearly as possible. Repeat 10 times. To make this sound correctly, the tip of the tongue flicks off the soft palate behind the top row of front teeth.

ARTICULATION EXERCISES

A stroke can leave a person with labored speech that is halting, breathy and even indecipherable. It was very difficult for Jo to say more than three words at a time because she could not manage her breath or remember the sequence of words. The goal of our initial speech and sound exercises was to break down the letters of the alphabet into individual sounds and learn how to pronounce these sounds clearly. From there we worked on words to phrases and finally to sentences.

Here are three suggestion when practicing these exercises:

1. Have client watch you perform the exercise as you emphasize the correct mouth movement and articulation.

2. Have client look in mirror and observe themselves as they speak.

3. Record your client's speech exercises and play them back. Jo was very surprised to hear what her voice really sounded like.

The following speech exercises work on strengthening and coordinating the vocal muscles and helps to develop vocal awareness. Certain words will help focus on certain areas of articulation.

To bring lips together, practice P, B, and M words.

Pat, peanut, pie, purpose, peace, point, pickle, principle, prime, print, pronounce, pump, pig, punch, press, pumpkin, pal. Bacon, bed, brilliant, bright, baby, bar, banjo, band, blueberry, book, beast, beauty, bean, benefit, babble, baboon. Mother, moth, mine, merry, might, more, meager, mental, mention, meaningful, measure, medic, mark, margin, maybe.

To bring lower lips in contact with upper teeth, practice F and V words.

Ferry, fight, figure, fat, free, fly, four, fine, fit, fever, fickle, feud, fetch, fiber, fig, field, fiddle, force, far, finger, fire, finite. Very, vine, vigor, vigilant, velvet, vacation, vail, valid, vampire, vanity, variation, vase, variety, vase, verb, vegetable.

For the tip of the tongue, practice TH, T and D words.

Thought, thin, they, thorough, thus, thwart, thymus, thunder, throttle, throw, thrust, thumb, thump, thorn, thread, thrive, ton, ten, time, tin, torrent, toggle, toe, tired, tiny, tip, tissue, temporary, toad, toilet, turkey, tomato, tool, train, tradition. Dab, dime, dinner, danger, darling, daughter, date, dark, dip, debate, dish, debrief, debit, declare, decline, deck, deep.

For the back of the tongue and the soft palate, practice K, G and NG words.

Kind, keep, knew, knap, knack, knight, know, knot, kefir, keel, kettle, kempt, kelp, knee, knowledge, kohlrabi, kite. Great, guy, giant, grub, graduation, grown, guide, guess, gray, grease, gratitude, green, grind, grocery, ground. Lung, bring, bang, hang, king, long, ping, swing, string, ring, sing, strong, young, longer, jungle, hanger, finger, hunger.

For soft palate, practice words that make the E sound.

Eagle, eager, east, even, event, easy, eat, ecology, effect, enough, eject, ego, either, electric, elation, elastic, eleven, elite.

To stimulate vocal cords, practice H words.

Habit, hackle, hack, haddock, hades, hail, honey, hope, hype, hoard, hand, happen, hard, heel, heat, hide, hobble, how, hole, hot, hounds, house, howl, horse, hub, husband, heather, heavy, heedless, horsepower, horror, hose, hospital.

For the back of the tongue, practice words which have "ack," "ake," "ig," or "og" sounds.

Black, acknowledge, track, back, backward, backtrack, crack, flack, fracking, cracker, jacks, hack, hijack, knack, lack, sack, packer, quacked, lake, take, fake, rake, make, shake, awake, bake, bakery, breaker, brakes, cake, cheesecake, drake, dressmaker, intake, keepsake, earthquake, namesake, pancake, fig, gig, pig, rig, big, swig, trigger, sprig, wig, earwig, brig, shindig, frog, bog, log, bogus, dialog, clog, dog, groundhog, hotdog, leapfrog, log,

For the front of the tongue, practice words that have "S and SH" in them.

Simmer, snake, sign, signal, slip, slot, several, slate, snow, supper, simple, snore, slight, sit, sigh, sing, song, soar, shimmer, shake, ship, shine, shout, shove, short, shot, shortwave, shovel, shred, shriek, shrewd, shoulder, show, should.

For a full mouth workout, say "buttercup," "rocket ship," and "organization." Repeat each word 5 times.

ACTIVITY: Vowels – A, E, I, O, U

Goal: To recognize and relearn the sounds of the vowels.

Directions:

1. Practice saying the sound of each vowel clearly. Repeat 10 times.

2. Practice the vowel sounds while exaggerating lip and jaw muscles.

3. The vowel "o" will work the open mouth. The vowel "A" will stretch the mouth and jaw open. The vowel "E" will stretch lips and cheeks. The vowel "U" will work the lips.

4. Practice the vowel sounds and hold as long as possible. (AAAAA, EEEEE, IIIIIIIII, OOOOO, UUUUU).

Sing the vowel sounds!

ACTIVITY: Alphabet Drill

Goal: To improve recall of alphabet and to imitate letter sounds.

Directions:

1. Use alphabet flash cards or write out the letters on an index card. Go through the alphabet and say each letter slowly and clearly. Have client repeat the letters after you.

2. Then have client say the alphabet without assistance.

4. Try singing the alphabet song. It helps with recollection.

ACTIVITY: Reading Word Cards

Goal: To improve reading and pronunciation of words.

Directions: Write out familiar words on an index card. Have your client read the words aloud.

ACTIVITY: Blending Vowels and Consonants

Goal: Distinguish and articulate sounds.

Directions: Say each sound to your client and have him or her repeat the sound back. Stress articulation and demonstrate how to make the sounds with your lips. Repeat each word group three times.

BA, BE, BI, BO, BUU
DA, DE, DI, DO, DUU
FA, FE, FI, FO, FUU
GA, GE, GI, GO, GUU
HA, HE, HI, HO, HUU
JA, JE, JI, JO, JUU
KA, KE, KI, KO, KUU
LA, LE, LI, LO, LUU
MA, ME, MI, MO, MUU
NA, NE, NI, NO, NUU
PA, PE, PI, PO, PUU
RA, RE, RI, RO RUU
SA, SE, SI, SO, SUU
TA, TE, TI, TO, TU U
VA, VE, VI, VO, VUU
WA, WE, WI, WO, WUU
YA, YE, YI, YO, YUU
ZA, ZE, ZI, ZO, ZUU

ACTIVITY: Consonant Blend Drills

Goal: Recognition and clear pronunciation of common blended sounds.

Consonant blends are groups of two or three consonants in words that makes a distinct consonant sound, such as "bl" or "sp." These can be very tricky to pronounce so patience and practice is the key. This is just a list to get you started. These blends can be at the beginning, in the middle or at the end of words. See if you can come up with your own consonant blends. Check out the thesaurus or online sites for ideas.

Directions:

1. Coach pronounces the constant blends and the client repeats.

2. Emphasize the beginning sound clearly to client.

3. Encourage client to pronounce the sound as clear and distinct as possible.

BL - black, blue, blight, blizzard, blarney, blame, blanket, blaze, blank, bleed, blend, bleep, blemish, blah, bladder.

BR - brand, brass, bread, break, breathe, breeze, brew, branch, brain, braid, brake, bride, breathe, breeze.

CH - charm, cheese, cheap, cheek, chicken, child, chili, chin, chase, chat, charm, chime, cherry, chess, chew.

CL - clash, classic, classify, clause, classroom, claw, clay, cleanse, clean, clear, clench, clever, clink, clarify, clamor.

CR - crab, crack, crackle, cradle, crafts, cranberry, crane, cranky, credit, crazy, create, crawl, creature, creek.

DR - drab, draft, dragon, drain, drama, drank, draw, drawer, dramatic, drum, drown, drunk, dry, drought.

FL - float, floor, flop, flip, flint, flow, flower, flu, flourish, flour, floss, flood, flag, flipper, florist, flood, flute, fly.

FR - fraction, fragile, fragment, fragrant, frail, frame, frank, frantic, fraud, free, freeze, frighten, friend, fret.

GR - grab, grace, graceful, gracious, grad, grade, gradual, graduate, grand, grandchild, grain, grant, grain, grapes.

PL - plaza, plea, pleasant, please, pleasure, pledge, plenty, pliant, pliers, plight, plug, plumber, pluck, plum.

PR - prairie, prance, pray, precipitation, precious, precise, precocious, predict, present, president, press.

SC - scam, scan, scandal, scanner, scapegoat, scar, scare, scarecrow, scarf, scarlet, scary, scathing, scatter, scarlet.

SK - skate, skedaddle, skeet, skein, skeleton, sketch, ski, skid, skill, skillet, skim, skip, skinny, skin, skipper, skirt.

SN - snag, snail, snake, snap, snapdragon, sneeze, sniper, snare, snarl, snatch, snazzy, sneak, sneaker, sneer, snip.

ST - steak, steam, stem, step, steep, stick, sticker, sting, stomach, stone, stool, stoop, stop, store, storm, story.

TH - these, those, them, thought, thank, thigh, things, think, therapy, thirsty, theatre, thirty, thrown, thin.

TW - tweak tweed, tweet, tweeze, tweezers, twelfth, twelve, twenty, twerp, twice, twiddle, twig, twilight.

TR - transmit, transparent, transport, trap, trapeze, trash, travel, tray, tread, treasure, treat, treble, tree.

WR - wrack, wrote, wrangle, wraparound, wreathe, wring, wrinkle, wrist, wristwatch, wrong, write.

ACTIVITY - CH & SH Consonant Blends

Goal: Distinguish two difficult sounds from each other (CH and SH).

Directions:

1. Go through the CH list. Repeat each word three times.

2. Practice the SH list. Repeat each word three times.

3. Alternate both the CH and SH lists together.

CH

Chalk, chain, challenge, chamber, champion, chance, charge, change, channel, chant, chap, chapel, chapter, chariot, charity, charm, chart, chase, chat, cheap, check, checkers, cheek, cheer, cheese, cheetah, chef, cherry, chess, chest, chew, chick, chicken, chief, child, chili, chime, chimp, chair, chin, china, chip, chisel, chocolate, choice, choose, chop, chore, chose.

SH

Shack, shade, shadow, shake, shall, shampoo, shamrock, shape, share, shark, she, sheep, shelf, shine, shepherd, ship, shirt, shock, shoots, shop, shore, should, shoulder, shuck, shut, shock, showers, show, shell, short, ship, shed, shower, shark, shave, shift.

ACTIVITY - Tongue Twisters

Tongue twisters certainly make the speaker stop and think of what they are trying to say as well as focus on making the correct sound. Try it yourself and see. This simple exercise is actually quite an effective one. Tongue twisters are excellent warmups for all the vocal muscles: lips, tongue and jaw.

When I introduced tongue twisters to Jo, I had to reduce the twister phrase to three or four words because she could not remember more than that. Over time, she was able to repeat five out of six words in the phrase. You can experiment with longer twisters if your client can handle the challenge. You can find online or you can make some up on your own!

Goal: To improve pronunciation in an entertaining way.

Directions: Start with shorter phrases and work up to longer ones. Read the phrase slowly and have client repeat. If memory is a problem, write out the twister and read aloud.

- A big black bug bit a big black bear.
- Betty beat a bit of butter to make a better batter.
- Friendly Frank flips fine flapjacks.
- Which wristwatches are Swiss wristwatches?
- A noisy noise annoys an oyster.
- Lovely lemon liniment.
- The lips, the teeth, the tip of the tongue.
- A box of biscuits.
- Six thick thistle sticks.
- Sally sells seashells by the seashore.
- A mellow, yellow fellow.
- Reading and writing are richly rewarding.
- Red leather, yellow leather.
- Peter piper picked a peck of pickled peppers.

MULTISYLLABIC WORD LISTS

Practicing words with multiple syllables help improve speech rhythm and breathe control. You can start with the simple two-syllable word list and work up to the five syllable or you can combine words from all the lists for practice. Practice ten minutes daily.

Two Syllable Words

baby, bacon, balloon, baseball, bedroom, bedtime, berry, body, bunny, butter, button, goodbye, bathtub, rabbit, neighbor, paper, pancake, pencil, people, pizza, popcorn, sleeping, toothpaste, pepper, ketchup, table, syrup, teacher, tired, toilet, closet, tonight, towel, doctor, dinner, Monday, Tuesday, Wednesday, Thursday, Friday, Sunday, reading, birthday, color, forehead, breakfast, finger, vacuum, farmer, cookie, weekend, music.

Three Syllable Words

basketball, bicycle, blueberry, broccoli, neighborhood, library, umbrella, principal, privacy, apricot, piano, potato, policeman, envelope, telephone, hospital, beautiful, computer, tortilla, screwdriver, tomato, chocolate, parking lot, spaghetti, spider web, dinosaur, dangerous, grandmother, grandfather, grasshopper, lemonade, tricycle, post office, fingernail, butterfly, slipper, video, vitamin, government, camera, category, gigantic, ladybug, coloring, sandwiches.

Four Syllable Words

anybody, obedient, celebration, librarian, discovery, roller skating, impossible, invisible, vegetable, appreciate, questionable, vice president, peanut butter, police station, apologize, supermarket, chocolate chip, temperature, television, calculator, elevator, alligator, escalator, thermometer, historical, motorcycle, dandelion, asparagus, congratulate, misunderstand, understanding, cauliflower, photographer, avocado, caterpillar, kindergarten, cooperate, conversation.

Five Syllable words

planetarium, personality, hippopotamus, denominator, potato salad, refrigerator, alphabetical, mathematical, disorganization, disagreeable, unquestionable, electricity, cafeteria, unforgettable, vocabulary, veterinarian, anniversary, university, California, congratulations, cooperation, communication, imagination, elementary, condominium, organization, curiosity, laboratory, auditorium, vegetarian.

LANGUAGE- BUILDING EXERCISES

ACTIVITY: Alphabet Game

Directions: Type or write each letter of the alphabet in list form with room to write a word next to it. Ask your client to name a word that begins with each letter of the alphabet.

Be sure to record the starting and ending time for this activity. This activity is a good way to generate words and show progress. Jo got to the point where she could name a word

for all but four letters of the alphabet! That was huge progress for her.

A....apple
B....bacon
C....cat
D....?

ACTIVITY: Rhyming Family Word Groups

Rhyme, like rhythm, emphasizes patterns, which is one way our brains organize information and makes it meaningful. It also helps identify family word groups that helps one understand language. Word families are groups of words that have a common pattern or groups of letters with the same sound. An example of a word family would be "et." Members of that word family include "let, get, met, set." Goal: encourage auditory awareness, vocal rhythm and pattern recognition.

Directions:

1. Have the alphabet written out (A-Z) in large letters for this exercise to use as a reference tool. Remind client that if they are having trouble thinking of a word, they can just go through the alphabet, letter by letter, until they come to a letter that forms a rhyming word.

2. Select a family word group to work with. Ask your client to think of as many words as they can that have the word pattern.

AIN - brain, chain, complain, explain, gain, grain, main, obtain, pain, rain, Spain, strain, train.
ACK - attack, black, crack, hack, jack, knack, lack, pack, quack, rack, sack, tack, track, whack.
AK - awake, bake, brake, cake, fake, flake, lake, make, quake, rake, sake, shake, snake, take.
ALL - ball, call, fall, gall, hall, install, mall, small, stall, tall, wall.

AN - ban, bran, can, Dan, Fan, man, pan, ran, scan, tan, van.

AT - bat, brat, cat, chat, fat, flat, gnat, hat, mat, pat, rat, sat, that, vat.

ASH - bash, cash, clash, crash, dash, flash, hash, lash, mash, rash, sash, smash, trash.

AW - claw, draw, flaw, gnaw, jaw, law, paw, raw, saw, slaw, straw, thaw.

AY - away, bay, clay, day, flay, gay, hay, lay, may, nay, okay, pay, play, ray, say, spray, stay.

EAT - beat, cheat, feat, greet, heat, meat, neat, peat, seat, treat, wheat.

EN - amen, Ben, children, den, glen, hen, men, open, pen, then, ten, when.

ELL - bell, cell, dell, dwell, farewell, fell, hell, sell, shell, smell, swell, spell, tell, well, yell.

EST - best, chest, jest, nest, pest, quest, rest, test, vest, west, zest.

ENT - bent, cent, dent, event, gent, lent, rent, scent, sent, spent, tent, vent, went.

IDE - bride, decide, glide, hide, pride, ride, side, stride, tide, wide.

IGHT - bright, delight, fight, flight, fright, height, knight, light, might, night, plight, right, sight.

ICE - dice, ice, mice, nice, price, rice, slice, spice, thrice, twice, vice.

ICK - brick, chick, click, flick, kick, lick, nick, pick, quick, stick, thick, tick, trick, wick.

IN - bin, chin, din, fin, gin, grin, shin, skin, sin, spin, think, tin, twin, win.

ING - bring, cling, fling, king, ping, ring, sing, sling, swing, thing, wing zing.

OG - blog, clog, dog, fog, frog, hog, jog, log, smog.

OT - blot, clot, cot, dot, forgot, got, hot, jot, knot, lot, not, plot, pot, rot, shot, slot, spot, trot.

OUT - about, bout, clout, out, lout, pout, scout, shout, snout, stout, trout.

OW - bow, blow, crow, flow, glow, grow, low, mow, row, show, slow, snow, sow, stow, throw.

UG - bug, dug, hug, jug, lug, mug, plug, pug, rug, shrug, smug, snug, thug, tug.

ACTIVITY: Common Phrases

Directions: Complete the phrase. Most of the time, it is the last word in the phrase that you are trying to get your client to say. Just experiment and have fun. You will be amazed to see how the brain remembers these common phrases even when you have not heard them in years! Here are a few examples to get you started. Plenty more can be found online.

1. Don't beat around the bush.

2. Close but no cigar.

3. Don't cry over spilt milk.

4. Don't look a gift horse in the mouth.

5. When it rains it pours.

6. Curiosity killed the cat.

7. Every cloud has a silver lining.

8. He was a Jack of all trades.

9. It's like finding a needle in a haystack.

10. Like father like son.

ACTIVITY: Synonyms & Antonyms

Working with synonyms and antonyms will increase your client's understanding of language. A thesaurus is a great tool for these exercises and others. Synonyms are words that share similar meanings with other words.

Direction: Ask your client, "Can you think of another word that means center?"

Word	Synonym
center	middle
damp	wet

hurry	rush
hear	listen
lost	missing
odd	strange
sad	unhappy
small	little
smile	grin
stay	wait

Antonyms. Antonyms are words that mean the opposite of other words. To do this exercise, ask your client, what is the opposite of big?

Word	Antonym
big	little
young	old
come	go
poor	rich
before	after
brave	scare
laugh	cry
healthy	sick
narrow	wide
boy	girl

Another way to use antonyms is to say a sentence and have your client say the same sentence using the opposite of the word.

Examples:

Coach: Here is a **large** apple.
Client: Here is a **small** apple.
Coach: That country is **above** the equator.
Client: That country is **below** the equator.
Coach: He was a **young** man.
Client: He was an **old** man.

SENTENCE BUILDING EXERCISES

PARTS OF SPEECH

Here are the basic parts of speech: adjectives, adverbs, conjunctions, nouns, prepositions, pronouns and verbs.

- Adverbs modify a verb, adjective, or other adverb (slowly, rapidly or quietly).

- Adjectives are words that modify a noun or pronoun (long, pretty, quiet or happy).

- Articles are a special category of adjectives. Articles include only: a, an, and the.

- Conjunctions join words in a sentence (and, but, or, nor, for, yet).

- Nouns name a person, place, thing, idea, or concept (Mary, London, turnip or freedom).

- Verbs are words that describe or show action or state of being (ran, jumped, wrote, and sang).

- Prepositions link a noun or pronoun to some other word in a sentence. Prepositions include: in, of, to, about, above, across, after, against, along, behind, below, beneath, beside, between, down, except, for from, in, off, on, onto, opposite, out, outside, to, toward, under, underneath, until, with, within, without, in and through.

- Pronouns are words that take the place of a noun. Examples: I, you, he, she, it, we they, me, him, her, it, us, them, those, this and that.

ACTIVITY: Fill-in-the Blanks with Verbs

Goal: To improve language and reasoning skills.

Directions: The simplest way to work with sentences is to do fill-in-the-blank exercises. Create your own fill-in sentences by looking for simple sentences in any type of printed material, select the verb and remove it. Then provide three verb selections that your client can choose.

Write the sentences down and have the client circle the correct choice. These exercises are on teaching websites and in learning skills workbooks. Encourage your client to select the verb that makes the most sense in the sentence. Some examples:

1. Let's (fly, ride, jump) a kite.

2. The puppy (barked, talked, laughed).

3. The man (jumped, walked, cried) over the fence.

4. The bird (painted, laughed, sang).

5. The man and woman (cried, screamed, climbed) the ladder.

6. The young man (drove, shot, paddled) the canoe.

7. The musician (threw, tied, strummed) the guitar.

8. The mailman (ironed, dipped, delivered) the mail.

9. You need a (hose, rake, hammer) to gather up the fallen leaves.

10. Pour some milk into your (spoon, cup, plate).

More Difficult:

1. I want to play outside, but it (is, are, am) raining.

2. This candy (is, are) too sweet to enjoy.

3. In fact, there (was, were) no final plans available at the meeting.

4. There (is, are) some paper on the desk.

5. The color of these roses (is, are) red.

6. Everyone in the class (is, are) present today.

7. All the furniture in my house (is, are) brand new.

8. The windows in the room (is, are) dirty.

9. Everyone (is, are) present at the conference.

10. There (are, is) some paper on the desk.

The purpose of these verb and noun exercises is to practice the cognitive skill of "reasoning," to determine which the most accurate answer is. Even though the exercise seems simple, there is an important cognitive process happening in the background as there is for all these exercises. As your client advances in ability, you can increase the difficulty of the multiple-choice answers.

ACTIVITY: Select the Correct Noun

Directions: Follow the same directions as above, only this time select the noun and remove it. Provide three noun selections that your client can choose. Some examples:

1. We wash our (hair, sofa, lamp) with shampoo.

2. We write with a (carrot, pen, shovel).

3. We wear a (dress, desk, potato chips).

4. There are many different kinds of fish in the (pantry, car, river).

5. The (church, theatre, restaurant) has good food.

6. When it is cold outside, I put on a (bathing suit, apron, jacket).

7. To mail a letter, I go to the (post office, library, gas station).

8. We cook on a (dishwasher, refrigerator, stove).

9. We put gloves on our (head, hands, feet).

10. We wear boots on our (feet, arms, head).

ACTIVITY: Complete the Phrase with a Noun

Goal: To encourage vocabulary, reasoning skills and auditory skills.

Directions: Read the phrase aloud and ask client to complete. Remember, there can be more than one correct answer. Have fun creating your own phrases.

We read a _____	We kick a_____
We sing a_____	We comb our_____
We open the_____	We ride a_____
We hit a_____	We row a_____
We climb a_____	We button a_____
We build a_____	We feed the_____
We mow the_____	We tell a_____
We paint a_____	We water the_____
We empty the_____	We dry the_____
We clean the_____	We eat a_____

Another variation of working with nouns is to have your client complete a familiar phrase with a common noun. Read the following phrases aloud and have your client complete the phrase.

A loaf of _____	A spoonful of _____
A piece of_____	A drop of _____
A bottle of_____	A dish of _____
A glass of_____	A pack of_____
A drink of_____	A quart of_____
A bag of _____	A head of_____
A pile of_____	A bar of_____
A bunch of_____	A swarm of_____
A box of_____	A jar of_____

ACTIVITY: Choose an Adjective

Adjectives are words that describe a noun (person, place or thing).

Goal: Increase understanding of sentence structure, word meaning and vocabulary.

Directions: Find simple sentences in grammar workbooks, magazines, online sources, or make up your own sentences. Have client read the sentence aloud. Then have client circle, underline or point to each adjective in the sentence that describes the noun.

If your client struggles with this exercise, use very simple adjectives: quantity (one, four) or colors (blue, green) or texture (soft, hard) or size (large, small) or shape (round, flat, square).

Examples:

1. The green leaves began to sprout on the tree.

2. She put on her red shoes.

3. The heavy bag was filled with clothes.

ACTIVITY: Building Sentences

Goal: To promote understanding of English language and sentence structure.

Directions: Every sentence has a subject (noun) and an action word (verb). It can be simple. The **girl sat**. It can grow in complexity by the addition of adjectives and adverbs. The **lovely** girl sat **gently on the couch.**

Continue to add on to a sentence according to your client's ability to understand. The lovely girl sat gently on the **old** couch in the **dark living room.** I usually do this sentence building exercise in several steps, using who, what, how, where and why questions as prompts.

1. Select a noun like dog.

2. Write out the sentence like this
The_____dog_____.

3. Ask client to identify or describe the **noun,** in this case, dog by giving an adjective such as brown, sweet, cute, etc. It can be helpful to ask:

What kind of dog?
Can you describe the dog?
What size is the dog?
Is the dog happy or angry?

Next, ask your client to describe what the dog did (verb). The dog **ran.** The dog **barked.**

Finally, ask client where the dog barked. (See list of prepositions). Did the dog bark **outside, inside, across** the street, **behind** the fence, etc.?

ACTIVITY: Understanding Nouns

Goal: Improve ability to name and describe common objects and their function.

Directions:

1. Show client an object or a picture of an object.

2. Ask them to name the object if possible. "What is this object called?"

3. Ask them to describe its use or function. "What is this object used for?"

4. Ask them to describe the object in terms of size, color, shape, weight, texture, quantity and age.

5. Using your client's answers, or your own, create a sentence describing object/ noun. Example: "It is a large, purple pillow to lay your head on."

ACTIVITY: Word Clusters

Goals: To improve memory, language and association skills. Sometimes called mind maps or word clouds, these are clusters of associated words surrounding the topic word in the center of the page. You can find blank templates on line or just make your own. This exercise is excellent for improving word retrieval skills because usually one word leads to another word. At first, your client may need help to associate the word with these other ideas. With practice, however, it gets easier. It encourages vocabulary development and word association skills. Here is an example of words associated with the topic word "*garden.*"

Directions: Pick a word and write it in the center of the page. Circle it. Have client find words that associate with the circled word. Draw lines from the circle word to the new word.

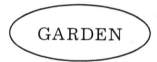

Dirt, shovel, dirt, seeds, grow, sunshine, rain, flowers, roses, vegetables, tomatoes, peas or food.

ACTIVITY: Spelling

Goals: To improve memory and language processing skills.

Directions:

1. Write two misspellings and one correct spelling of a word. Example: *EQWAL, EQUAL, EQUALL.* Have the client select the correctly spelled word by either circling, underlining or pointing to it. If needed, tell the client what the word means. Then, have client use the word in a simple sentence. *Please cut the pie in equal portions.*

2. Select simple words from a thesaurus and ask your client to repeat word and then spell it and finally use in a sentence. Begin with simple words and increase difficulty according to the client's abilities.

ACTIVITY: Alphabetizing

Goals: Develop organizational and sequencing skills and to improve memory.

Directions: Present your client with a list of printed words on index cards or cut words from newspapers or magazines and ask the client to arrange them in alphabetical order. Alphabetizing from A to Z is the simplest version of this exercise. You can increase the difficulty by using words that have the first two or three letters the same such as tribe, tribute, and triangle. You can alphabetize the months of the year. Use a thesaurus or dictionary to generate words.

ACTIVITY: Word Search

Goals: Practice focus, concentration, and visual recognition and language skills.

Word retrieval is the ability to recall known words that are stored in long-term memory. Word search books are an excellent way to practice this skill. You can use either adult or children's books, depending on your client's abilities. Word search and word scramble puzzles are offered free of charge on line at many of the educational or teacher sites. Simply select your own words and the program scrambles them into a pattern and prints the puzzle with an answer key. One good site is www.atozteacherstuff.com.

To make your own, simply write a selected word such as *NOSE* and surround it by other letters. The purpose is to have your client find the hidden word. The more letters that are added to the word, the harder the challenge. Start easy and progress in difficulty. Example: *YUINOSEGHU*. It might help to let client know what category the words are in like food, body parts, animals, etc.

Activity: Unscramble the Words

Goals: Practice focus, concentration, and visual recognition and language skills.

As the coach, you can vary the difficulty of this exercise depending on how you scramble the letters. If you keep the first two or three letters in the proper place and then scramble the other letters, it will be easier to unscramble. A very easy scramble for the word *plate* would be *plaet*. A harder scramble would be *tlpae*. Just select any word and mix up the letters to create a scrambled word exercise. You can also find online programs to create scrambled word worksheets.

1. You can create scrambled sentences by going through magazines and cutting out the words in a phrase, headline, or sentence and then mix them up. Ask your client to put them in the correct order. If the font is too small for the client to read, type sentences on your computer with a large font, print, then cut up and scramble.

2. Another fun thing to try is a magnetic poetry board! Select words that will form a sentence then, scramble them on the board and have your client make up a sentence from the pile of words. To avoid confusion, be careful not to put too many words down on the board at once.

ACTIVITY: How Many Words Can You Form?

Goals: Practice focus, concentration, memory and language skills.

Directions:

3. Select a word with lots of letters and ask your client to create as many words as

possible from the given word. Be sure to write down that word on the paper as well as the new words your client forms from that word.

4. Ask, How many words can you form from the word *rehabilitation*? Examples: habit, bear, hat, rat, tin, lab, hill.

Another variation of this exercise is to use scramble tiles. Have your client spell words with scrabble or word tiles. Scrabble is an excellent word generating game. Remember games can always be adapted to meet your client's needs. It just takes a little imagination and patience.

CATEGORIZATION EXERCISES

Categorization is the ability to group words or objects into groups based on their shared characteristics. This type of activity encourages flexibility in thinking as well as developing skills in comparison as to why things are alike or different. The following is a list of categories that you can use. You can incorporate these categories in any of the above exercises such as word scrambles, alphabetizing, spelling, etc.

Types of Animals
Body Parts
Days of Week
Things that are round
Kitchen Items
Forest Animals
Types of clothing
Furniture
Types of Food
Sports
Types of Tools
Things that Fly
Toys
Transportation
Facial Expressions
Musical Instruments

Famous Singers
Things made from Metal
Fruit
Types of Containers
Vegetables
Flowers
Desserts
Holidays
Things to Drink
Types of weather
Occupations
Things worn on the head
Things found in the ocean
Birds

ACTIVITY: What Does Not belong? What Belongs?

Goals: Encourages reasoning, visual processing, association, and categorizing abilities.

Directions: Present your client with a list of words or images from magazine or therapy cards. Ask them Which one **does not belong** with the others? An example would be book, table, and chair. You can also ask your client to find the words or images that **do belong** together. To increase the difficulty of this exercise, ask your client to explain why these words do or do not go together.

ACTIVITY: Sorting Images or Objects

Goals: Develop categorization and motor skill abilities.

Directions: Instruct your client to sort the objects into piles of similar objects.

You can use just about anything for this exercise if it has enough quantity and variation such as coins, colored paper clips, cut-out images, therapy cards, playing cards, marbles, stamps, coupons, sports cards, etc.

ASSOCIATION EXERCISES

The following exercises involve finding out how two or more objects are similar or dissimilar to each other. The objective is to identify the important features, or attributes, of these objects. Some common basic attributes are color, size, shape, composition and function. Baseballs and footballs are similar in that they are both balls, both thrown, and are both objects used in games. The differences are in size, shape, color, weight, materials and function.

ACTIVITY: Same and Different

Goal: To improve the ability to associate.

Directions: Have two objects or two images on the table. Ask your client to observe both images carefully. Remind them to consider their characteristics or attributes (size, color, shape, function). Ask your client to explain the *difference* between the two objects in detail. Then explain the *similarities* between the objects.

ACTIVITY: Image Hunt

Goal: To improve ability to follow instructions, association and visual processing skills.

Directions: Select a category like things *that are round* or *things that are green* or *things you can eat,* etc. Ask your client to look through magazines and find images that belong in each category.

ACTIVITY: What Am I thinking?

Goal: To improve visual and auditory processing, reasoning and language skills.

Directions: Describe an object and see if your client can guess what it is. To make this exercise easier, I would have five images of objects on the table: wheel, plate, ball, ruler, compass and cookie. Then I would describe the object I am thinking of. "It is round, and it is used to find direction." This game can be increased or decreased in difficulty according to your client's skill level. Flashcards that display images of objects are wonderful to use. You can find images to use in magazines too.

ACTIVITY: What is it?

Goal: To develop reasoning, analyzing skills and memory.

This game is similar to riddles. Although it is a game, it can be very, very challenging for those who have difficulty naming objects.

Directions: Describe an object with as much detail as possible. What is something that is alive? Its color is green, and it grows everywhere and needs to be cut often?

The answer is grass. You can modify the difficulty of this activity by showing images of several objects and then have your client guess which one you are describing.

ACTIVITY: What Goes With What?

Goal: To develop categorizing, pattern recognition and analyzing skills.

Directions: Create a list of words or collect images and have client find matches for the words or images that belong together.

ACTIVITY: How Many Things Can You Name That Are...?

Goal: To develop language, memory and association skills.

Directions: Ask your client to name objects or point to images that are green or long, or sharp or hot or flat, etc.

PATTERNING EXERCISES

Exercises that involve patterns help the brain organize information and anticipate what will come next. There are pattern worksheets that you can download at educational online sites such as www.Kidzone.com or www.mathworksheets4kids.com. Patterns include sequences that repeat, alternate, grow or decrease in the sequence. Patterns can include numbers, colors, letters, shapes, and more.

Patterns can also be three dimensional with the use of objects such as a deck of cards, marbles, coins, buttons, stamps, etc. You can create your own patterns from the following examples and vary the patterns from easy to hard depending on your client's ability. Just remember, in a repeating pattern the item or number predictably. A "growing" pattern is a pattern in which the numbers *increase* in a predictable way. A "decreasing" pattern is when the numbers *decrease* in a predictable way. Music is also a great way to practice pattern recognition.

I found that when Jo had difficulty determining a pattern on a worksheet that had different images, I would demonstrate the same pattern with colored pencils and crayons. Coins would also work well for creating patterns. Just use your imagination. You can create three-dimensional patterns by using objects you find around the house like ear swabs, toothpicks, silverware, assorted nails, paper clips, etc. Encourage your client to create their own pattern once they have become proficient at recognizing different patterns. Make a game of it by having both you and your client create and complete patterns for each other!

Examples of Pattern Sequences:

A, B, C, D, E…
Aa, Bb, Cc, Dd…
A B A B…
AA BB AA…
A B C A B C…
A B B A B B…
AAA BB AAA…

NUMBER PATTERNS WITH "RULES"

1, 2, 3, 4… (Number increases by "1" each time)
1, 3, 5, 7, 9… (Number increases by "2" each time)
5, 10, 15, 20… (Number increases by "5" each time)
10, 9, 8, 7… (Number *decreases* by "1" each time)
100, 90, 80… (Number *decreases* by "10" each time)
1, 2, 4, 8, 16… (Number doubles itself each time)

FOLLOWING DIRECTIONS EXERCISES

You can be creative and have fun with this exercise. Demonstrate the instructions and have your client mimic your actions. Then have client follow directions, without a demonstration. For even more challenge, write directions down and have client read and perform independently.

Two-Part Instructions

- Touch your nose and your chin.
- Raise your hand and wave.
- Wink and smile.
- Wiggle your thumb and touch your knee.
- Point and make a fist.
- Close your eyes and stick out your tongue.
- Open your mouth and cough.
- Smile and shut your eyes.
- Wrinkle your nose and scratch your head.
- Shake your head and point your finger.
- Raise your foot and stomp.
- Straighten your leg and shake my hand.
- Point to your ear and then your forehead.

Three-Part Instructions.

- Point, smile and wave.
- Scratch your head, open your mouth, and make a fist.

- Tap your shoulder, touch your knee, and stomp your foot.
- Touch your nose, your mouth and your hair.
- Smile, shake your finger, and wink.
- Smile, rub your hands, and clap.
- Raise your left hand, wave, and snap your fingers.
- Point to the ceiling, the floor and me.
- Touch your knee, your elbow, and your chin.
- Shrug your shoulders, and stomp your left foot.

COGNITIVE CONVERSATIONS

Do not underestimate the importance of simply having a conversation with your client. Answering questions stimulates discrimination and memory skills. Questions require the brain not only to remember and retain information but also to articulate a timely and accurate response. If possible, ask questions that require a response other than "yes" or "no." Come up with questions that your client can answer and increase difficulty according to their ability.

ACTIVITY: What Is Happening In This Picture?

Directions: Select an image from a book or magazine or even a photograph that depicts a person in a scene. Ask your client what is going on in the picture. You can ask questions such as:

1. What is the person wearing?

2. What is the person doing?

3. What do you think the person is thinking?

4. How do you think the person feels?

5. What would you like to ask this person?

6. Why are they doing what they are doing in the picture?

7. Where is this person going?

8. What do you think will happen next? ?

9. What colors do you see in this picture?

10. How does this picture make you feel?

ACTIVITY: What Does This Statement Mean?

Directions: Pick one of the following sentiments or statements and discuss it with the client. Ask them what they think the statement means. Do they agree or disagree with it? Can they recall an event or situation where this statement makes sense? Can they rephrase the statement in their own words? Use the statement as a springboard for conversation. Have fun with this activity and see where it leads!

1. Beauty is in the eye of the beholder.
2. Out of sight, out of mind.
3. As one door closes, another opens.
4. Home is where the heart is.
5. Leave tomorrow until tomorrow.
6. The best things in life are free.
7. Better to wear out than rust out.
8. Give a man a fish, and he will eat for the day. Teach him to fish, and he will eat forever.
9. His eyes are bigger than his belly.
10. Too many cooks spoil the broth.

ABSTRACT THINKING ACTIVITIES

Just as cognitive conversations exercise the brain, abstract thinking involves the brain's higher thinking skills. To think abstractly one needs to be able to conceptualize, organize their thinking, understand multiple meanings, recognize patterns, problem solve and think both critically and creatively. One way to encourage abstract thinking skills is to think aloud and ask questions about what is happening in either a real situation or an imagined scenario.

Directions: Think aloud with your client about something that is happening now or recently. This could be something from current events, a news story, television show, you-tube video, or a recent conversation or event. A passage from a story or lyrics from a song or poem would also work well. This helps your client recognize analogies or "this is just like that" reasoning skills.

Understanding the Event: Client talks about what they think is happening in a situation or scenario to the best of their ability. Coaches can coax clients by asking what, when, who and why questions. Coaches can also share their own interpretation.

Making Connections: Ask the client if they can remember a similar event or circumstance in their past. You can assist your client by asking:

Do you remember a time when you experienced something similar?

Did you ever meet a person like that? Can you think of other examples?

Is there anything in your life that is similar to this situation now?

Alternative Perspectives: Questions to ask: Are there other ways to think about this? How might other people think or feel differently?

What If: Discussion is encouraged by coach asking, Can you imagine another ending for this scenario? What do you think might happen as a result?

Making Connections: Discussion is encouraged by coach asking, What can you learn from this scenario?

Evaluations: Discussion is encouraged by coach asking questions. How can we decide if this is a good thing or not? Do you think this is a good thing ? Why or why not?

Reasoning: If this is true, what else can we assume to be true?

HANDWRITING AS A COGNITIVE TOOL

The practice of handwriting is a powerful activity. It awakens muscle memory, improves manual dexterity and exercises hand and eye coordination. The goal behind handwriting is to practice the proper shape and form of individual letters and numbers. This can either be by printing or writing cursive. I chose handwriting as a means of achieving four goals for Jo:

1. Increase fine motor skills in her non-dominant hand.
2. Improve her ability to record her thoughts and feelings in written form.
3. Exercise tactile and visual processing.
4. Improve her memory and concentration.

Quite a lot to ask from such a simple activity! We started by focusing on improving her hand and eye coordination and finger dexterity. Jo began by tracing letters from grade school handwriting books. This exercise challenges someone with vision problems because the lines can appear blurry. One way to help is by highlighting the letter so it is easier to see and trace. Jo was faced with both vision difficulties and learning how to use her weaker non-dominant hand for writing.

A stroke can sometimes leave survivors with a condition known as post-stroke movement disorder, which involves rapid involuntary motions of flexion (tightening) and extension (stretching). Jo had to deal with twitches and tremors that came on suddenly in her left hand when she was holding something or reaching for something. Naturally, these involuntary movements presented challenges for almost every activity from drinking water, to picking up an object, to holding a paintbrush. We did our best to work around them. Sometimes, we even used them to our advantage as in the case of drawing and painting where spontaneous and curious little wiggly pen strokes added interest to the artwork. Unfortunately, it did not work that way when it came to handwriting, in which case, the clearer the line or stroke, the better.

It is important to try a variety of writing tools and see which gives the most control. There are adaptive pens that slip over the fingers, fat pens and pencils, markers (thin and thick), crayons, chalk and regular sized pens and pencils. We tried them all and with varying success. We started out with the chubbiest implements and worked our way to regular sized, easy-flowing pens and pencils. Pencils have a medium drag (resistance across the page). Ballpoint pens have less resistance and felt tip markers have even less. If you want to enlarge the diameter of the writing tool, you can purchase foam pencil grips or buy pens and pencils with enlarged grips. Experiment and see what works best.

Finger Position. Holding the writing tool properly can provide a challenge especially for clients who are using their non-dominant hand. The correct position forms a tripod with the thumb, index and middle fingers. Be sure that your client holds the pencil so that they can see what they are writing.

Paper position. Right-handers need the upper right-hand corner of the page to be higher. Left-handers need the top left-hand corner to be higher. Attach the paper to a clipboard, slant board or taped to a sturdy piece of cardboard. It helps to put non-skid shelf liners on the working surface. I used this material to provide stabilization for almost all our activities. An inclined writing surface such as a slant board or easel encourages the client to write with wrist and arm in an extended position. Use large binder clips to hold pages in place as well. If the writing tablet or journal is wire bound, be sure that the spiral is on the top, so that it does not interfere with the hand. You can get a left-handed writing tablet, if your client is using that hand.

Lined paper provides a challenge of staying within the lines, while unlined paper makes writing in a straight line difficult. We tried both. Often, I would draw the lines so that there was more space for Jo's letters, which tended to be quite large. Almost all activities and exercises will need a certain amount of adaptation.

Lighting is another factor to consider. It is important that the writing surface is well illuminated. If your client is writing with their left hand, the light is on the right or slightly in front of the writing surface. If the client is right-handed, the light should come from the left and slightly in front. This avoids shadows across the paper.

Tracing is a good pre-writing activity. If your client has difficulty with handwriting, provide them with letters and shapes to trace. You can find tracing forms online, or you can buy tracing paper and make your own worksheets. I found that when Jo traced letter forms or shapes and then attempted them on her own, she had a better understanding of what needed to be done and did better.

If you do not want to invest in handwriting books, then you can draw lines, circles and other shapes on plain white paper with and have your client trace over them with a darker shade of ink. You can use the computer to print out practice pages. Do be sure that the letters or shapes are large enough. Jo and I tried dot-to-dot drawings and mazes. Whichever practice you use, I would recommend dating these pages so that you can visually record your client's progress and provide encouragement.

Cursive writing adds an extra cognitive punch because your client has to recall how to shape the letter and also how to string the letters together as well as how to determine the space between letters. Re-learning to write with a non-dominant hand that has never written before is frustrating and requires patience and practice. It is a good idea as a coach, to jump right in and practice with your non-dominant hand alongside your client!

Exercise Warmups.

Before beginning a handwriting or drawing session, I had Jo do finger and hand warmups. Here are some exercises we did:

- Squeeze fingers into a fist and release. Repeat ten times.

- Turn wrist palm up and palm down. Repeat ten times.

- Touch each finger to thumb. Repeat ten times.

- With fingers flat on table, lift each one up. Repeat ten times.

- Stretch fingers wide apart and hold for 5 seconds. Relax. Repeat ten times.

- Twirl wrist. Repeat ten times.

- Touch right hand to left shoulder and left hand to right shoulder. Repeat ten times.

- Shrug shoulders. Repeat ten times.

- Roll shoulders forward and backward. Repeat ten times.

ACTIVITY: Writing Letter Forms

Directions: Have client practice alternating printed and cursive styles of writing. See which style they prefer and practice that one until they become proficient. Practice writing:

1. Rows of straight letters like Roman capitals: I, J, K, L, M, N, T, R, K, V, W, X, Y and Z.

2. Rows of rounded letters like lowercase: m, n, a, b, c, d, e, g, h, p, q, and o.

3. Rows of lowercase cursive letters that have connect to each other in to one long continuous line: e, l, s, f, p, g, u and o.

4. Practice writing words within a large rectangle or square. Then decrease the size of the rectangle and square, so the client has to write smaller to fit the word inside.

5. Practice writing the days of the week, months, names, words and sentences.

OTHER ACTIVITIES TO DO AT HOME

Card Playing

A deck of playing cards provides many opportunities to practice cognitive skills. They are wonderful because they are cheap and easy to take with you wherever you go. They not only provide entertainment but also exercise the skills of attention, dexterity, concentration, sequencing, association, pattern recognition, and association, to name a few!

1. For a motor dexterity exercise, have the client take a card from the top of the deck and turn it over into another pile. This provides an opportunity to practice "grasping" skills and wrist turning. Another variation of this activity is to have your client practice dealing out the deck of cards equally into two piles. You can increase the challenge by increasing the number of piles. At the end of the exercise, have your client count out the cards that are in each pile. Encourage your client to increase their dealing speed if they can.

2. Have your client sort the deck according to black and red colors.

3. Have your client sort the deck according to suits (clubs, diamonds, hearts and spades).

4. Lay down a variety of colored cards and have client count how many red and how many black cards are on the table.

5. Lay down the number one to ten cards using only one suit. Have your client put cards in numerical order.

6. Try playing card games like solitaire, war and go fish.

Working with Money

Coins are excellent for practicing cognitive skills such as attention, memory and problem solving. Play money provides an opportunity to work with paper denominations.

1. Lay a mix of quarters, nickels, dimes, and pennies on the table. It is best to start with six to 12 coins and increase the number of coins according to your client's ability. Have your client sort the coins according to value by putting them in a container. Have four cups, jars or another suitable container for this purpose.

2. Make the activity more challenging by having your client close their eyes and pick out a certain coin such as a dime by touch.

3. You can also use coins to help your client improve math skills. Ask them to give you a certain amount such as 45 cents or 23 cents.

4. You can also have the client add up the total amount of coins on the table.

Writing and Reading

1. Write emails or letters.

2. Make lists such as grocery lists or lists of objects on a table or in a room.

3. Look at recipe books and copy down favorites.

4. Complete dot-to-dot activities.

5. Do mazes.

6. Color in coloring books.

7. Doodle.

8. Use magnetic words and letters to make sentences or phrases.

9. Listen to books on tape and discuss the story.

10. Watch movies with subtitles.

11. Read newspaper and magazine stories in print or digital versions.

12. Keep a journal.

13. Compare ingredients between two similar canned or boxed products. Which ingredients are different?

Time Money and Numbers

1. Practice making change.

2. Practice writing checks.

3. Practice math skills by adding up the year's utilities bills.

4. Practice time awareness with clocks and watches. Set alarms and turn them off.

5. Practice dialing on the phone.

6. Plan a food budget. Go through food advertisements and circle items to add to list. Write down the price of each item. Then add up the total.

7. Collect US quarters, dimes or pennies by year.

8. Keep a calendar of daily activities.

9. Practice keeping a real or pretend budget based on your client's ability to handle financial transactions.

Memory

1. Go through photograph books and ask the client to recall who was in the photo and what was happening at that time. Play online video games and "brain" games.

2. Play games like Pictionary, solitaire, Sequence.

3. Sing songs.

4. Recite poetry.

5. Watch movies and TV shows and discuss characters, series of events and storylines.

Household Chores

1. Practice sorting objects like silverware.

2. Empty dishwasher.

3. Put food away in the refrigerator.

4. Sort or alphabetize bills.

5. Put stamps on envelopes.

6. Do some tabletop gardening: water plants, plant seeds and transplant flowers.

7. Wash or rinse dishes.

8. Sort laundry and put in washer and dryer.

9. Set the table or clear away the dishes.

10. Make juice from frozen concentrate.

11. Practice using household items like blenders, toasters, the dishwasher, remote control, etc.

Arts And Crafts

1. Try craft activities like scrapbooking, stamping or model building.

2. Use decorative hole punches on card stock paper and thread yarn through hole.

3. Use decorative stickers.

4. Playdough or Thera putty.

Games

Games are a fun way to learn and they do not feel like work! They are an opportunity for the stroke client to interact with others. Look for games and activities that work on the following skills: manual dexterity, concentration, word recall, visual acuity, memory, language and cognitive flexibility. If you find that a game is too hard for your client, adapt and modify the game. Take away the pressure of time or use easier questions, eliminate some rules, or buy the junior version of the game. Educational game shops offer a great selection of innovative games and activities.

Jigsaw Puzzles
Word Puzzles
Crossword Puzzles
Dice Games
Legos
Lincoln Logs
Marbles
Jenga

Card Games

Go Fish
War
Slap Jack
Concentration
Solitaire
Phase 10
Old Maid
SET

Board Games

Checkers
Pictionary
Connect Four
Battleship
Scattergories
Scrabble
Upwords

Game Shows

Jeopardy
The Price Is Right
Wheel of Fortune

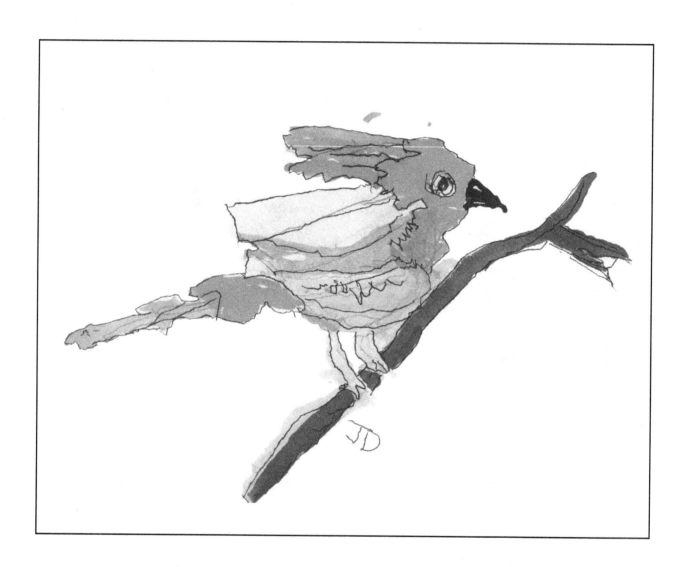

CHAPTER SEVEN

AS THE BODY HEALS

The limits of the possible can only be defined by going beyond them into the impossible.
—Arthur C. Clarke

As her cognitive coach, I worked with Jo to help her improve communication and cognitive skills, which and did not include physical therapy exercises. Although I was not involved in any of the activities that worked her major muscles: legs, arms, and trunk, I did do massage and exercises with her affected hand. There were several physical therapists and occupational therapists that she saw over the years for those exercises. When therapy sessions ended with the therapists, she continued doing them at home with the assistance of her husband and other caregivers.

Physical therapy exercises were not part of my cognitive program. I am a firm believer in the supervision and guidance of a physical therapist during recovery. Home exercises should be under the direction of a medical professional. They need to explain how to do the exercise correctly. You never know what harm can come from doing an exercise improperly, especially when the client cannot communicate clearly about pain and discomfort! However, there are some safe and commonsense suggestions you can do at home to help your loved one or client on their physical recovery path.

- Massage affected body parts gently to improve circulation and stimulate sensory awareness.

- Encourage loved one or client to move their limbs, even if they are in a wheelchair. They can shift positions, stretch, reach for something imaginary, turn their heads, etc. They can also do self- massage and stretch the fingers of their affected hand.

- Drink plenty of fluids.

- Eat a healthy and nutritious diet.

- Encourage purposeful movement having your loved one or client control as much as they can in their environment. Purposeful movement would include controlling operating the wheelchair, reaching for objects, washing their face, brushing their hair, and getting dressed on their own.

Physical Symptoms That May Be Present After Stroke

Pain is an unfortunate symptom of stroke and it can be constant and unrelenting. Jo suffered from many of the symptoms on the below list. It was amazing that she had energy left for our sessions! Managing her pain was an extreme challenge for her husband. Pain is a complicated matter and should be discussed with the family physician or rehab professionals. It is essential to discuss any issues of dizziness, which is a common side effect of stroke with medical professionals.

It is a good idea to explore all options for pain management, including alternative or complementary medicine such as relaxation techniques, acupuncture, etc. Pain can affect the patient's ability to maintain balance for movement and walking activities. Ask the stroke patient if they have problems seeing. Is there ringing in their heads? Do they feel nauseous or weak? See if they can describe when the dizziness begins. Is it first thing in the morning? Make notes of the stroke patient's comments as you go through their daily actives, being alert to the moments that they complain about their dizziness. Be sure to share this information with the family or medical professionals.

The majority of the following physical symptoms most likely will be present in the early stages of post-stroke. Some may continue for a long time afterward as the patient recovers, and others may extend through the lifetime of the survivor. Each body will heal at its rate. The important thing is to address each of these issues and find the best medical professional to help. The important thing to remember is NEVER GIVE UP HOPE!

- Exhaustion
- Pain
- Dizziness
- Shaky movements in non-affected limb
- Weak grip and inability to grasp objects
- Exhaustion
- Viral Infections
- Vision difficulties
- Problems with spatial orientation
- Swallowing difficulties
- Urinary tract infections
- Nausea due to medications
- Tight, painful muscles
- Spasticity. This affects the arm or hand by making the muscles stiff so that they contract (shorten) and form into a tight fist.
- Headaches
- Bladder control
- Exhaustion

- Shoulder subluxation
- Muscle fatigue
- Foot drop
- Central pain syndrome
- Weak trunk strength
- Gait dysfunction
- Muscular atrophy

RECOVERY AFTER STROKE

Rehabilitation Environment There is some current research that suggests that the environment in which rehabilitation takes place could play a significant role in the patient's outcome. The environment includes physical setting, the methods used to deliver recovery, the type of intervention, intensity, and the knowledge, skills, and attitudes of the staff. There are several different rehabilitation environments.

Inpatient rehabilitation facilities. These are usually part of a hospital or clinic. They are designed for patients who need twenty-four-hour care by medical staff. Here they will receive physical and cognitive therapy from specialists. The patient stays here for several weeks and sees a variety of therapists and specialists during their stay.

Outpatient units. They can be part of a hospital or clinic. The patient spends several hours a day receiving intensive focused physical and cognitive therapy and returns home at the end of the day.

Skilled nursing facilities. Medical staff care for the patient and assist with the activities of daily living (ADL), and light to moderate therapy.

Home environment. Therapy programs are done at home by the primary care provider with or without follow-up treatments by medical professionals.

How long does stroke rehabilitation last? Rehabilitation will depend on the severity of the stroke, what areas of the brain are damaged, the age of the survivor, responsiveness to therapy, and other related complications. The program of rehabilitation will change along the way to reflect the needs of the patient. I think it is essential that a stroke patient have a manageable amount of stimulation each day, along with exercise. If most of the patient's days are spent in one or two rooms of the house, then that does not offer enough visual and cognitive stimulation. It makes sense to provide different experiences in other areas of the house, yard and beyond. Going for drives, going shopping, and any activity that requires the stroke patient to interact with the public and relearn social skills is helpful. Such stimulation might even affect how much effort they put into their presentation, posture, and attempts at communication.

Rehabilitation Delivery Methods

Research and clinical trials evaluate the effectiveness of different delivery methods of rehabilitation therapy. Some standard and cutting-edge methods include:

- Constraint-induced treatment, also known as forced-use therapy, involves restricting the use of an unaffected limb while only moving the affected limb through a range of activities.

- Task-specific training to facilitate activities of daily living or other relevant motor tasks.

- Range-of-motion therapy uses exercises and other treatments to help lessen muscle tension (spasticity) and regain range.

- Motor skill exercises to help improve muscle strength and coordination.

- Mobility training may include learning to use walking aids, such as a walker or canes, or braces to stabilize and assist in supporting body weight while relearning to walk.

- Functional electrical stimulation involves using electricity to stimulate weakened muscles, causing them to contract.

- Robot-mediated therapy (RMT). Robotic devices can assist in movement.

- Body weight-supported treadmill training (BWTT). Treadmill walking with body weight partially supported.

- Pharmacotherapy such as Botox injections.

- Transcranial magnetic stimulation (TMS) is a noninvasive method used to stimulate small regions of the brain using a magnetic field generator or "coil" that placed near the head.

- Brain-computer Interface (BCI). An EEG reads the brain waves as the patient concentrates on moving their hand and then sends an impulse in the electrodes stimulating the arm's muscles.

- Transcutaneous neuromuscular electrical stimulation is the use of an electric current produced by a device to stimulate the nerves for therapeutic purposes.

- Stem cell research.

- Patient-centered therapy where the patient is encouraged to have more responsibility and motivation in their recovery, such as goal setting,

- Complementary medicine treatments, such as massage, herbal therapy, acupuncture, mental imagery, water therapy, semantics, yoga, body movement, chiropractic, and more.

REHABILITATION PROFESSIONALS

Physical Therapist (PT)

Physical therapists are health care professionals who help individuals maintain, restore, and improve movement and activity. They also work with large muscle groups and focus on walking and balance.

Occupational Therapist (OT)

Occupational therapists tend to work predominately with the small muscle groups above the waist up, such as arms, hands, fingers, etc. Occupational therapists focus on helping patients perform the activities of daily living such as bathing, tying your shoes, or buttoning your shirt.

Speech-Language Pathologist (SLP)

Speech-Language Pathologists evaluate, diagnose, and treat speech, language, communication, and swallowing disorders.

What To Look For In A Rehabilitation Professional

Jo was very fortunate that her husband was an intelligent and resourceful health advocate for his wife's recovery. He educated himself on the subject of stroke, its treatments, and his wife's prognosis. He kept accurate logs on his wife's health symptoms, exercise regimes, diet, and medication schedules. He wanted to communicate effectively with doctors in determining the best care for his wife. He looked for the best practitioners and was not timid about asking hard questions and demanding satisfactory results from them. Jo's husband did all the right things a primary caregiver should do. He provided a clean, safe home environment, nutritious meals, and helped her with bathing, dressing, and toileting activities. He managed her catheter and trachea and was quickly on top of any complications with either device

Most importantly, he consistently remained positive and encouraging about his wife's recovery and surrounded her with people who shared his optimism. I learned many things from this amazing individual. He showed me that it was okay, and even necessary, to change health practitioners if you are not satisfied with the relationship you have with them. Sometimes the reasons for dissatisfaction are that the physician or therapist does not give you enough time to ask questions during the appointment. Even more importantly, they might not listen to what you are saying or take your observations seriously. Jo's husband never accepted "less than" from the physicians and medical professionals. Neither should you!

I have nothing but the most profound respect for physical therapists. I think those that go into this profession are a special breed of people who have good people skills, along with strong communication and problem-solving skills. They are usually highly knowledgeable and passionate about their field of expertise. I believe that the relationship one has with their health practitioner is so meaningful that I think it warrants some further mention here. The following is a list of traits I would look for in a therapist. You may have some others you want to add. So, before you go shopping for a physical or occupational therapist, consider the qualities they should possess. The following is a checklist that you can use.

- Exhibits confidence and professionalism.

- Considers the whole person and not just the condition.

- Excellent listener and answers your questions.

- Flexible thinking skills.

- Gives information in a clear, concise manner and welcomes questions.

- Gives feedback on the patient's progress.

- Stays on top of the latest research and techniques in the profession.

- Works well with other medical professionals.

- Receives positive referrals from other patients.

- Encourages patient involvement and ownership in the rehabilitation plan.

- Provides "homework" for at-home exercises.

- Provides positive reinforcement.

- Can provide patient access to state-of-the-art exercise equipment.

Rehabilitation Goals

One of the main goals of physical therapy exercises is to increase the patient's **range of motion** (ROM) while decreasing pain, swelling, and stiffness. The range of motion is how far a person's joints can move in all directions. Range of motion exercises includes bending, flexing, twisting, swinging, reaching, pushing, pulling, and stretching. The physical therapist will determine what activities are needed to improve ROM, and they will be performed both during a therapy session and assigned as homework.

You may hear the therapist use the terms: *flexion or extension* to describe the exercise. *Flexion* is the action of bending limbs and joints closer together (e.g., making a fist). *Extension* is the opposite of flexion. It increases the angle that the limbs and joints are from each other (e.g., knees are extended (straight) when standing, flexed when sitting). Here are standard terms that most physical and occupational therapists use to describe the range of motion:

Passive Range - Involves someone (caregiver or therapist) moving the patient's limbs for them because the patient is unable to perform the movement. This is important in the early stages of stroke to keep the limbs flexible and to prevent them from tightening or shortening. Example: when a therapist holds your arm gently and moves it in a circular motion.

Assistive Range - Involves external assistance or support to complete motion. The therapist or caregiver will assist the patient as they attempt to move their limbs. This will help them achieve the full range of motion that they cannot do themselves. It is the first stage where the patient is actively involved.

Active Range - Patients will move their limbs independently without external assistance.

Besides improving range of motion, here are other rehabilitation goals that are common to stroke survivors and for anyone who has a weakened or damaged physical condition.

Besides improving range of motion, here are some other rehabilitation goals:

Increasing Core Strength - improves spine stability and strength.

Improving Balance - makes it easier to move about to stand, walk, etc. and reduces the risk of falls.

Increasing Flexibility - keeps muscles relaxed and joints limber.

Increasing Endurance - improves heart and lung fitness, reduces fatigue, and increases energy.

Increasing Strength - increases muscle strength, so it is easier to do everyday things like climb stairs, get up from a chair, and carry groceries.

If you are working with a client on physical exercises, a physical therapist should advise you of the duration and intensity as well as the proper body mechanics for each activity.

They can show you ways to avoid pain, dizziness, or overstretching in your client. They should also instruct you on how to work with your client without injuring yourself or the patient. It would be best to have the physical or occupational therapist watch you as you perform these activities on your client. It is a perfect time to ask questions and receive input. Another advantage of having a relationship with a physical therapist is that they are familiar with emotional issues that arise from physical rehabilitation, such as fear of falling or fear of failure. They can offer suggestions or give the patient a referral to another professional who can assist.

Designing Purposeful Movement Exercises

Isolated or repetitive exercises focus on specific body parts to improve flexibility, strength, and range of motion to that body part. They are essential for rehabilitation. Purposeful movement or "functional" exercises incorporate several muscle groups to accomplish a function or purpose, such as the activities of daily living. (ADLs). The current philosophy in the rehabilitation field is that the most effective exercises are those that assist the patient in managing their activities of daily living (ADLs). Exercises either can contribute to a functional movement (getting out of bed), or they can lay the groundwork towards completing that function (rolling from side to side). It gives the patient a sense of purpose and a feeling of accomplishment as they strive toward a specific movement goal. The larger picture starts to come together. If the patient can practice moving a dust cloth across a table, or reach for utensils out of a drawer, they will see how a functional movement brings them closer to independence.

I encourage you to see what type of activities you can do with your loved one or client to help them feel they are accomplishing tasks, however small, and participating in the household. Encourage your client to take pride and ownership in the particular task. Even if the client cannot perform all the steps in the task, let them do what they can, and offer assistance with the rest of the steps. Make adaptations and come up with compensatory strategies if needed. If the stroke survivor used to love to cook, have them measure ingredients, stir batter, add cut up ingredients to a bowl, etc. First, determine the steps to the activity, then consider what assistance your client will need to accomplish the action and then go for it! Be sure to make the activity fun and lighthearted. Here are some suggestions:

Household Tasks

- Sharpen pencils manually. Alternate hands or try an electric sharpener.

- Dust furniture in the house to practice arm extension, flexion, and circular turns.

- Put postage stamps on envelopes.

- Fold dish towels.

- Practice pulling open draw handles and knobs with both affected and unaffected hands.

- Empty and fill the dishwasher.

- Put food items away in refrigerator and shelves.

- Sort laundry into piles

- Fold socks into balls.

- Fold scarves.

- Sort jewelry items, cosmetics, office supplies, etc.

- Water plants.

- Fill up animal dishes.

- Sort mail.

- Turn off light switches at night.

- Lower blinds, if within reach.

- Turn on and off the TV remote.

- Practice making phone calls.

- Fill up birdhouses with seeds.

- Water the yard or garden with a hand-held hose.

- Put dirty clothes in the hamper.

- Brush lint off clothes.

- Alphabetize folders or bills, magazines, index cards, whatever.

- Plant seeds in seed containers.

EXERCISES AND ACTIVITIES FOR MOTOR SKILL PRACTICE

- Putting stickers on and pulling stickers off the paper.

- Typing on a computer keyboard.

- Cutting cloth or paper with scissors.

- Using a glue stick to adhere magazine images on paper to create collage.

- Coloring with templates.

- Pen drawing with a Spirograph.

- Removing caps from pens.

- Pick objects out of a container and sort in piles.

- Putting on makeup or face cream.

- Sorting cards from a deck of cards.

- Playing games like checkers and dominoes.

- Stringing beads.

- Pressing objects with thumb.

- Squeezing objects.

- Twist and turn lids on jars.

- Open and close plastic containers.

- Twist and turn can opener.

- Use a staple punch.

- Use a decorative punch to make shapes in paper.

- Pick up marbles and small objects between index finger and thumb.

- Pass crumbled paper back and forth between both hands.

- Moving beans from one container to another.

- Putting pegs in a pegboard.

- Using rubber bands to exercise fingers.

- Stacking pennies--challenging!

- Stacking wood or plastic blocks.

- Playdough--stretch, squeeze and shape the play dough into different shapes.

- Finger Painting.

- Tapping fingers to music.

- Marble shooting.

- Turn cards over and lay in neat piles.

- String beads.

- Work on puzzles.

- Practice buttons and zippers.

- Squeeze toothpaste from a tube onto a toothbrush.

- Mazes and dot-to-dot drawings.

- Writing.

Coach with Compassion

Work with your client's present abilities and make the most of where they are in the recovery path. It is essential to understand that the only REAL thing you and your client have is the PRESENT moment. As important as it is to remain hopeful and to work hard for a future of increased mobility and cognition, it is more important to understand what the patient CAN achieve right NOW!

A motivated patient will accept the responsibility of their healing, and they will continue to challenge themselves daily, stepping higher and higher up that mountain. If they tumble, they can pick themselves up and start again. Their belief that they can participate once again in the world will drive them to incredible heights.

AIM FOR WHAT CAN BE BUT FOCUS ON WHAT IS!

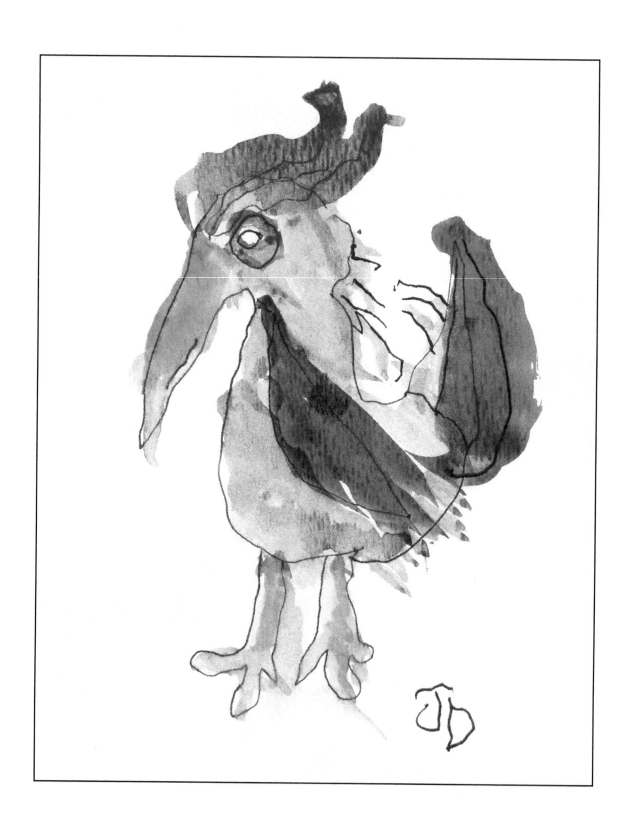

CHAPTER EIGHT

ART AND THE BRAIN

Art washes away from the soul the dust of everyday life. —PABLO PICASSO

Art, like music is a "whole brain" experience. It lights up many different parts of the brain and provides a great cognitive workout. As a practicing artist, I know the cognitive demands art requires especially in thought flexibility, decision-making and creative thinking. Art provides opportunities to use your problem-solving skills every time you correct mistakes or change direction. Art strengthens your visual spatial ability to process information visually. This includes recognizing patterns, understanding space, shape and form, and making associations. Art is a wonderful eye and hand coordination activity.

I chose art activities hoping they would provide Jo some distraction from her pain. I knew from personal experience that art is an excellent distractor when it comes to physical and emotional pain, and even boredom. Most of the time Jo told me her pain diminished or that she had forgotten about it while she focused on her art activity. Drawing and painting activities proved to be everything I hoped they would be and more. They were two of Jo's favorite activities to do, despite her being able to use only one hand.

Over the years, as Jo progressed with drawing and painting activities, I was amazed at the powerful effect they had on her. Not only did they give her an outlet for creative expression, but they also gave her a sense of self-accomplishment. Her brightly framed watercolor prints covered her house and family and friends enjoyed them. I was especially thrilled to see how doing artwork was helping Jo with the higher functioning skills: following instructions, making decisions, and solving problems. Her concentration was improving, and she was beginning to observe, reflect, and correct her work. Art was an incredible brain stimulator for her!

I would recommend doing art for anyone wanting to improve their creative and critical thinking skills. Drawing encourages us to think creatively and critically at the same time, activating both the left (logical and words) and right (creative and images) hemispheres of our brains.

Creative Thinking

- Creative thinking asks the questions: What could be? What if?

- Creative thinking is about pattern recognition and seeing how things relate to each other (association), including items that, at first glance, may not have anything in common.

- Creative thinking is about putting things together, related or unrelated, to form something entirely new.

- Creative thinking is not a linear path, but it usually keeps the whole picture in mind.

- Creative thinking encourages us to be flexible and come up with more than one solution to a situation or problem.

- Creative thinking fosters a sense of independence and playfulness, along with an adventurous taste for making discoveries.

Critical Thinking

- Critical thinking asks the questions: What do we know? How do we know it? What do we need to know?

- Critical thinking is how we observe, inquire, analyze, interpret, synthesize sequence, reflect, and evaluate information to make a decision or come to a solution.

- Critical thinking usually follows a linear process that goes from point A to point Z. The inquiry process is an example of critical thinking.

- Critical thinking is about following systematic procedures and directions.

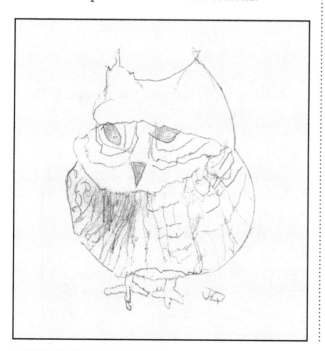

- Critical thinking is about using deductive reasoning to predict an outcome or draw a logical conclusion.

Benefits of Drawing

Most people recognize drawing as a kinesthetic and tactile exercise that improves eye-hand coordination. However, another benefit of drawing is that it helps us make sense of the world around us. It helps us make sense of it through patterns, shapes, and interconnections. As we draw, we learn about distance, size, and perspective.

Drawing encourages one to "see" what they are looking at. It requires the skills of observation and concentration. It does not matter whether that image is real or from the imagination. Either way, if we want to render a suitable likeness of an image, we must concentrate on that image, observing shape, line, contrast--all the details. For example, if you decide to draw a picture of a leaf on a tree branch, you must first distinguish that single leaf from all the others and focus on it exclusively. When you focus on the shape, shadings, contour, and lines of the leaf, you will see it as you have never seen it before.

Since drawing requires concentration, it can be a very meditative experience as the mind quiets itself down and focuses on the task. Music is a beautiful addition to a drawing session. Turn on some Mozart, Bach, or something similar that promotes a soothing, peaceful, and relaxed state of mind.

Drawing can take the "edge" off things by keeping your mind off what is bothering you and thereby being an excellent distraction from pain and depression. Being in a relaxed state encourages the release of positive brain chemicals like serotonin, dopamine, and endorphins into the bloodstream. These brain chemicals elevate your mood and can enhance new learning because a relaxed mind learns better!

Designing Art Activities to Achieve Cognitive Goals

While the art activities challenged Jo's ability to follow directions, they were also helping her retain information as well as take in new information. She was increasing her visual processing skills (taking information in from her eyes). She was learning to recognize patterns, make associations and understand the relationships of space between shapes. Art lit up Jo's brain and gave it a great brain workout! In addition, she was increasing the strength of her fine motor skills and learning information through her body (kinesthetically).

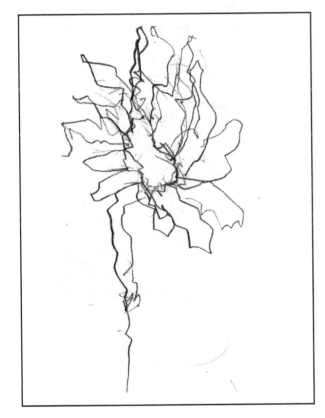

I would demonstrate the drawing goal several times before Jo understood and remembered the directions. Since Jo was not able to determine what the next step was, I had to give several drawing examples and repeat the directions often during the activity. Sometimes, it was necessary to focus on breaking down the image into "parts." It helped her recognize the relationship between things. We worked on shape and pattern recognition and reproducing the images as accurately as possible. To do this, she had to understand how to space objects adequately. The stroke had affected her visual field, so this was a challenge. At this stage, learning was through continuous repetition and example.

Doing a drawing or painting demonstration imparts valuable information to your client. It not only shows the steps involved to achieve the desired outcome but also provides an opportunity to learn how to spot mistakes, erase, and start over. It is okay to make mistakes, and it is even better if you can learn from them. Whenever Jo spotted her mistakes and then attempted to correct them, was exciting. This was a huge advancement from not knowing she had made a mistake to fixing it without advice from another. I believe motivation played a role in this as well.

Hand Warmups

Be sure to check with your doctor or physical therapist before attempting any exercise in this book!

Vary the number of repetitions according to your client's tolerance and ability.

- Squeeze fingers into a fist and release. Repeat 10 -15 times.

- Turn wrist palm up and palm down. Repeat 10 -15 times.

- Touch each finger to thumb. Repeat 10 - 15 times.

- Lay fingers flat on the table. Lift each one. Repeat 10 - 15 times.

- Stretch fingers wide apart (hold for five seconds) bring together. Repeat 10 - 15 times.

- Twirl wrist in both directions. Repeat 10 times.

Always be sure your client or loved one understands what the goal is that they are attempting to achieve. Do not assume that your instructions are always understood.

- Define the tools and resources needed for the activity (paper, pens, crayons, glue, lighting, etc.).

- Determine what limitations are present and make adjustments that will ensure successful completion of the activity.

- Demonstrate the activity in simple steps. Speak slowly and clearly.

- Show a finished example of the activity. Be cautious not to overwhelm your client.

- If the client is one-handed or using their non-dominant hand, demonstrate the activity using your non-dominant hand.

- Repeat directions as often as is needed.

- Allow the client to proceed with the activity independently. Offer assistance only if requested or to keep the activity on track.

- Be sensitive to how the activity is proceeding and make objective observations. What appears to be working and what doesn't?

- Are limitations in motor skills affecting the process?

- Implement changes when necessary. Change position, lighting, or the materials used, anything that might improve the overall activity.

- Ask for feedback. Be sure to encourage the client to stop and take a moment to look at their work and make assessments. Are they accomplishing the desired objectives? Will they get to where they want to go from where they are now? If not, what needs to be changed? Encourage the client to come up with his or her solutions.

- Always be supportive and encouraging. Point out what is working well. Avoid any negative comments about their progress.

- Manage the element of time. Be alert to exhaustion or frustration and take a break from the activity, if needed.

- Record your observations about the process so you can better select appropriate activities that are not too easy or too difficult.

- Always find something positive to say about your client's finished work.

- Lift wrist up and down (hammer motion). Repeat 10-15 times.

- With the arm straight, have client bend their elbow to shoulder and back. Repeat 10 - 15 times.

- Touch right hand to left shoulder and left hand to right shoulder. Repeat 10 - 15 times.

- Shrug shoulders. Repeat 10 - 15 times.

- Roll shoulders forward and backward. Repeat 10 - 15 times.

Select the following art activities in whatever order works best. Some people will be able to move quickly through the exercises, while others may need to do the same exercises or variations of it several times. Experiment with these exercises and try others. The goal is to find activities and exercises that provide cognitive challenges and help increase motor dexterity. Just about any art activity will accomplish this. I have offered a few ideas to get you started. If your client enjoys doing art, there are many, many websites, books, videos, and more to use as resources. Check out the education and art sites online, and visit your local craft store for more ideas.

INTRODUCTION TO DRAWING

Materials Needed:

Slant board or easel
Tracing paper, watercolor paper and drawing paper
Skid-proof surface or shelf liners
Standard set of drawing pencils and erasures
Colored pencils, crayons, chalk, crayons
Watercolor paints and brushes

PRE-DRAWING ACTIVITIES

1. Practice drawing vertical and horizontal lines.
2. Practice drawing curly or wavy lines.
3. Draw a square and ask your client to divide the square into four equal portions using intersecting lines. Repeat with different size squares. As performance improves, make the division more demanding. For instance, ask for six or nine squares created by intersecting lines.
4. Practice drawing a page full of circles.
5. Provide dotted outlines of shapes or figures and have the client fill in the shapes.

ACTIVITY: Recognizing Shapes in Images

Recognizing shapes helps to identify and organize visual information.

Directions: Find magazine images that are large enough so that the basic shapes can be seen easily (square, rectangle, circle, etc.).

1. Ask your client to find all the circular objects in the picture, then all the squares, rectangles, triangles, and diamonds, etc.
2. Have your client outline the shapes with a magic marker and name the shape as they are outlining it.
3. You can make a game of it by awarding "points" for every shape that is spotted. This is a good way to gage progress.

ACTIVITY: Magazine Collage

Collage is an enchanting way to be playful and creative. It can be used as a tool for self-reflection and self-expression. Its charm lies in its simplicity of materials: scissors, magazines, paper and glue. No previous artistic experience is required. One simply begins.

Directions:

1. Have a collection of cut-out magazine images and words that are ready to use.
2. Have client randomly select images and words that they are drawn to or that evoke an emotion.
3. Play music such as Bach, classical or piano music during the session.
4. Have client place cut out images and words on a sheet of sturdy paper. Encourage client to move the images and words around until they are satisfied.
5. Glue images in place.
6. Encourage client to talk about their collage if they feel comfortable doing so. They can also journal write about this experience.

ACTIVITY: Drawing Geometric Shapes

This activity helps with the organization of visual information and eye-hand coordination Basic geometric shapes to try are: square, rectangle, triangle and circle.

Directions: Give client a blank sheet of paper and a drawn example of a geometric shape.

1. Ask client to draw a geometric shape of their choosing.
2. Continue by drawing all the above geometric shapes.
3. When finished, have client circle their best images.

More Advanced:

Have your client practice drawing things that have obvious geometric shapes. Good examples are birdhouses (square house, triangle roof, circle opening); birds (oval or circle body, rectangle or leaf-shaped wings, circle head and smaller circle for eye, and triangle for beak); pine tree (triangle for tree, rectangle trunk); flower (circle center, rectangle or oval petals, rectangle stem, oval leaves).

ACTIVITY: Tracing Images and Objects

Tracing can help with hand-eye coordination, muscle memory and focus and special awareness. It's an important dress rehearsal for drawing! One can trace most any simple image or flat object. If using two-dimension images to trace, be sure to anchor the tracing paper over the image with tape or binder clips.

Directions: Have client practice tracing the following:

- Drawn images. Look for simple shapes without too much detail.

- Flat stones. Use stones of varying shapes and sizes.

- Hands. Trace own hand or another's hand.

- Alphabet. Trace upper and lowercase letters. Trace cursive writing.

- Geometric forms.

- Plastic or metal lids.

- Household objects.

ACTIVITY: Coloring

Directions: Use crayons or colored pencils to color an image in a coloring book. Start out with simple images and advance to more detail. Choose pictures according to your client's skill level and interest. Jo and I used coloring books that featured fashion dresses from the 1940's and 1950's which we both enjoyed. She also used watercolor paints in these books. Coach or client can also draw their own images to color if they want. Coloring pages are excellent for tracing too. Just attach tracing paper over the page with tape or binder clips.

ACTIVITY: Learning To Shade with Crayon or Pencils

This is an excellent tactile exercise for developing awareness of pressure and direction. You may find it helpful to tell your client what they want to hear is a "swooshing" sound as they shade with the pencil or crayon. This exercise is more challenging than one may think as it works on fine motor areas such as pressure, speed, and position.

Directions: Have your client hold their crayon or pencil at a 45-degree angle to the paper and begin to shade an area. Explore the difference between light and heavy pressure.

ACTIVITY: Color Groups

This activity gives practice at understanding and remembering directions as well as an opportunity to practice sequencing, categorizing and decision-making skills. It is also very relaxing.

Directions:

1. Mix a box of crayons into a pile.
2. Ask our client to sort the crayons according to color (all the yellows, greens, etc.).
3. Then have them choose a color pile and sort all those crayons from lightest to darkest shades.
4. Starting with one color group have client select the lightest crayon from that group and color a square or rectangle on the paper. Then select the next crayon that is a bit darker than the first and shade with that one, directly below or next to the first color.
5. Progress through all the color groups from lightest to darkest shades.
6. Try this with colored pencils.

ACTIVITY: Draw Organic Shapes, Squiggles, and Doodles

This exercise is a relaxing one that helps reduce stress, improve concentration, and increase muscle memory and motor skills. This free-form type of drawing focuses on shape, form and space. Anything goes with this exercise. Just let the pen, pencil or colored marker flow and have fun. This is a good activity to do while listening to music!

ACTIVITY: Drawing Patterns

This exercise helps with pattern recognition. It stimulates concentration and visual thinking skills. Pattern drawing repeats a shape or form in a consistent manner one after another, in a row, to create a unified pattern.

Directions: If your client cannot come up with their own ideas, draw or provide several pattern examples for them to choose. Letters and geometric shapes work well.

//// \\\\ //// \\\\ //// \\\\

<<<< >>>> <<<< >>>>

cocococococococococo

ACTIVITY: Draw Stick Figures

This is a simple way to draw the human figure. The focus is on drawing the basics of the figure in in the most basic forms: rectangle, circles, egg-shapes and spheres. This exercise can helps the drawer understand body positions, proportions and movement.

Directions:

1. Draw an oval-shaped head.
2. Draw a line for the neck.
3. Draw the torso. This can be a simple line or it can be a square or pillow-shaped form.
4. Draw a short line for the hips that

extends slightly from the end of the torso.

5. Draw two legs and add a simple shape for feet.
6. Draw a line for the shoulders that extends slightly from the top of the torso.
7. Draw two arms coming off the shoulders and add a simple shape for hands.

To increase difficulty, draw the stick figure in action poses: running, jumping, sitting, bending, etc.

ACTIVITY: Blind Contour Drawing

Directions: Without looking at their paper, have your client draw the outline of an object, which can be anything, even their opposite hand or your hand. Remind them to use just their eyes to "trace" the lines of the object without looking at their paper. This exercise can produce amusing results! It is a common exercise for beginning art students.

ACTIVITY: Partner Drawing

When Jo was having difficulties understanding how to draw an image, we took turns drawing the image together. This can be a fun activity. The results can be quite amusing and interesting!

Directions: Have an example of the image already drawn, so the client knows what the goal is.

1. The coach begins by drawing the head.
2. The client draws the neck.
3. Coach draws the shoulders.
4. The client draws the chest to the waist.
5. The coach draws one leg.
6. The client draws the other leg.
7. Coach draws one foot.
8. The client draws the other foot.
9. Coach draws one arm.
10. The client draws another arm.

Variations:

Do a partner drawing of a face.
Do a partner drawing of a scene together.
Color or paint the final image if desired.

Continue taking turns until the drawing is complete. After finishing, ask your client:

What they enjoyed most about the activity.
What was the most challenging?

ACTIVITY: Gestural Drawing

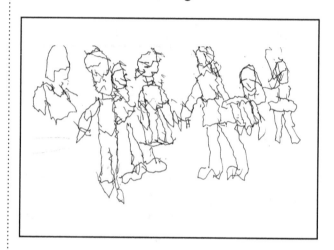

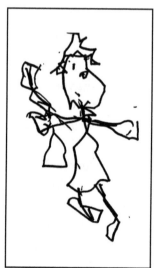

Gesture drawing explores the form and movement of an object in space, usually a human figure with quick energetic lines. It is different from stick figure drawing because a gestural drawing fills in the human form with details. A successful gestural drawing will capture the sense or feeling of the shape or

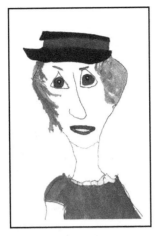

scene. It also emphasizes emotions.

Gestural drawings are an excellent way to show cognitive and motor skill progress. Whenever your client feels like they are not making any progress, it is good to bring out

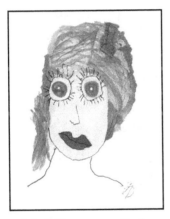

examples and let them see their progress. Jo put much detail into her gestural drawings emphasizing body poses, clothing, hair and facial expressions.

Gestural drawings usually become more precise and expressive as the client gains

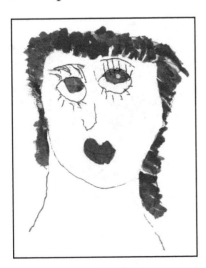

more skill, both in drawing and visualization. It is interesting to note how the illustrations can reflect physical, cognitive, and emotional states. Gestural drawing is also a perfect technique to use for an art journal which is a great form of non-verbal communication.

ACTIVITY: Targeted Drawing

This activity will involve sustained attention, discernment, decision-making, spatial awareness, and perception. The defining features are those features, shapes, and symbols that are prominent or distinctive. The goal is to copy an image as close as possible to the original image. This exercise can range from easy to difficult.

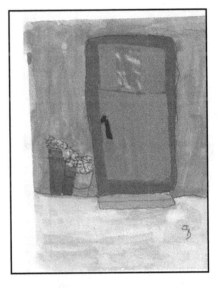

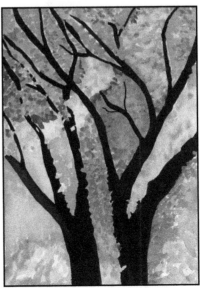

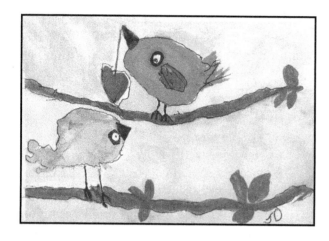

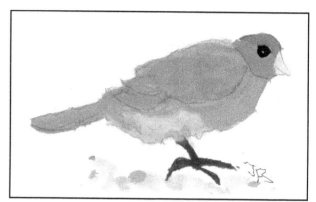

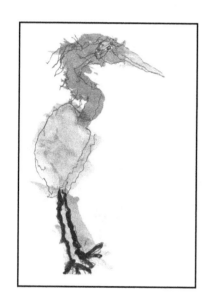

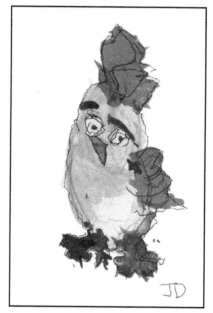

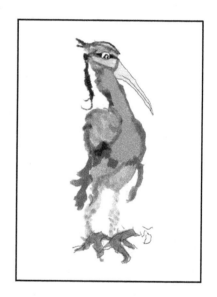

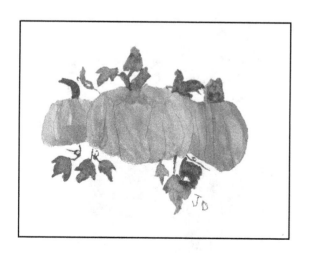

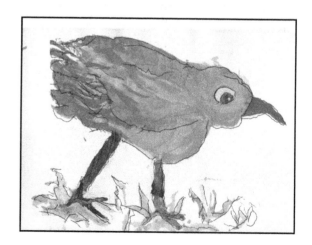

ACTIVITY: Draw or Paint a Figure

Directions: Have your client draw or copy images of people doing things. Encourage your client to draw all the body parts, including face, neck, hands and feet. The following are Jo's examples. She had great fun drawing and designing fashion for her "little women." Notice the details she gave her figures.

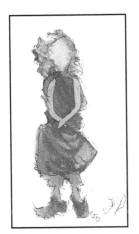 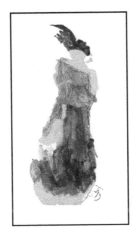

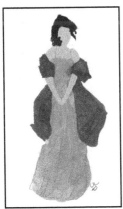 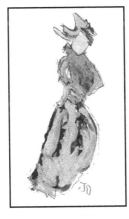

I was amazed at the creativity Jo put into each costume. She usually had an online image to copy and that got her started. She added her own creative interpretations which were wonderful. Jo had an innate ability to pick harmonizing colors. She put attention into detail showing the fold lines and hints of movement in the dresses. I believe that at this point in our journey, Jo was exercising the following cognitive skills simultaneously attention, visual processing, spatial, discernment, decision-making, problem-solving, reflection, self-correction and creative thought. I believe this was a pinnacle point in Jo's cognitive journey.

ACTIVITY: Drawing Birds to Emphasize Geometric Shapes

Birds are a great subject to draw. Basic bird images include: oval or egg shapes for the bird's body, a circle for the bird's head, a half circle for the wing, a small circle for the eye, a triangle for the beak, etc. I think there is an excellent value in focusing on geometric shapes such as the circle, square, and triangle as they are the basic shapes of everything that makes up everything. Jo's drawing successfully accomplished the goal.

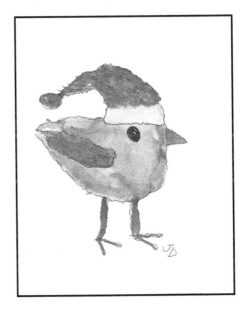

PAINTING

The art component of the program was expanded with the introduction of painting. Up until that point, my main goals were getting Jo to focus, maintain attention, understand directions, and improve her fine motor skills. Now, as our painting exercises increased, Jo would need to improve her decision-making, problem-solving, reasoning and creativity skills.

The painting style that we used emphasized a loose and energetic line flow that worked with Jo's abilities as well as limitations. The spasms that sent her hand across the page would produce squiggly lines that resulted in defining her style.

ACTIVITY: Mixing Watercolor with Water

Directions:

- Have client squeeze drops of watercolor paint onto a paper plate or plastic palette.

- Use paintbrush to dip into water and mix with paint until the paint is a smooth consistency. Less water will yield stronger, thicker color. More diluted paints will yield lighter colors.

- Practice doing long paint strokes with different sized and shaped brushes.

- Add more water to the paint to practice watercolor washes, which are very transparent layers of color. Work from dark to increasingly lighter washes.

ACTIVITY: Watercolor Resist with Crayons

Directions:

- Select a crayon and draw designs on white paper.

- Then paint over the crayon with a watercolor wash (thinned down paint) revealing the wax designs.

ACTIVITY: Painting with Sponges and Q-tips

Directions:

- Fill a palette with different watercolors and have the client dip a wet sponge into the colors.

- Dab sponge on white watercolor paint to create textures and designs.

- Try doing the same thing Q-tips to create dots of color. Several Q-tips can be tied together with a rubber band to create a cluster effect.

ACTIVITY: Painting Flowers for Fun and For Improving Motor Skills

Directions:

- Select a small # 4, 6, or 8 round brush. Dip the brush in black paint.

- Demonstrate what happens when the brush is held on its point (standing) and what happens when most of the brush is (sitting) on the paper. The standing line will be thinner than the sitting line. The amount of pressure on the brush will also make a difference in the weight or thickness of the line. It requires good motor control to control the brush.

- Instruct your client to hold or "stand" the brush on its tip and continue to hold it there as they move the brush across the paper to form thin lines.

- Practice these lines in both directions (vertical and horizontal). It requires reasonable motor control.

- Then practice laying the brush on its side to form the petals as in Jo's example.

The following are lovely examples of Jo's flowers. They show her ability to draw thin lines, sponge paint, outline, use Q-tips for flowers, and use her creativity!

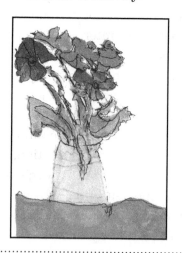

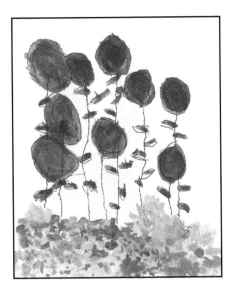

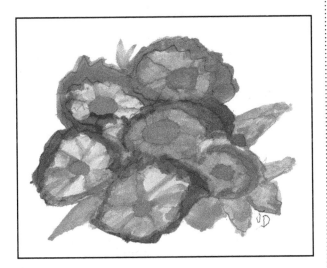

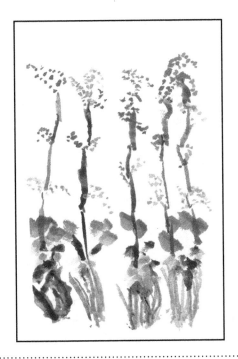

ACTIVITY: Bird Collage

This exercise was a lot of fun for both Jo and me. I wanted to present an activity that involved words, shapes, and new skills, such as gluing and cutting.

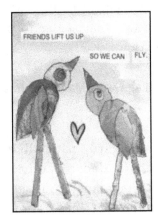

Directions:

1. Do a light watercolor wash for the background.
2. Paint foreground elements like a grassy hill, or patches of grass or flowers.
3. Set paper aside to dry.
4. Paint sheets of watercolor or shelf paper a variety of colors. Just spread color everywhere on the paper. You can use prepared decorative paper or even magazine pages.
5. Let the painted paper dry thoroughly.
6. Using a plastic or cardboard template, cut out the shapes of the bird's body from your decorated papers. I used a large oval for the body, a circle for the head, a triangle for the beak, a leaf shape for the wing, rectangles for legs, and small circles for eyes.
7. Use a glue stick to adhere the cut images to the paper.
8. Position a large oval (body) down first.
9. Do the same for twhe head, then wing, legs, and finally eyes. Use two circles for the eyes.
10. Once the images are glued on background, look for words to support the images.

11. Cut out inspirational or humorous words from magazines or print them out from the computer.
12. Glue words to background. The client may need assistance with the cutting and gluing processes.
13. Coat the entire picture with a Modge Podge or other sealer to preserve the artwork.

ACTIVITY: Collage with Magazine Images and Words

1. Select a sturdy paper like watercolor paper or cardboard for the background.
2. Sort through magazines and have your client cut out images that appeal to them. If needed, give assistance cutting out images.
3. Have your client select words that appeal to them at the same time they are looking for images.
4. Have the client arrange images and words on paper and glue them in place. Provide as much assistance as needed.

ACTIVITY: Daily Art Journal

The art journal is for personal expression. It is a safe place for your client to express whatever they would like to draw, whether it is abstract, figures, designs, etc. After the activity is finished, you can ask your client how they liked the activity before moving on to something else.

1. Find a blank drawing book with a spiral binding. Encourage your client to draw or paint whatever they want for approximately 15-20 minutes. Provide a choice of media to use pencils, pens, markers, etc. Be sure to date each page.
2. When they are finished, ask your client to turn to a blank page and write a few words about what they drew. This could be a paragraph or two, some simple phrases, or just words. Allow about 15 minutes for this exercise. This is optional.

Other Art Projects

There are many ideas for art and craft projects in craft stores. Select those that support your client's cognitive and physical abilities. Feel free to experiment with different art projects. The following are just a few ideas:

- Create words and designs with stamps and stamp pads.
- Paint plastic sun catchers.
- Paint wooden cut-outs.
- Papier Mache.
- String beads.
- Adult coloring books.
- Sticker books.
- Draw and color with stencils.
- Spirograph art.
- Draw mandalas.
- Paint small boxes, birdhouses, and other wood or paper forms.
- Stamping.
- Work with polymer clay.

*

Remember to always treat art as a fun and relaxing activity. Even while your client is having fun, their brains are working hard, and they are becoming more proficient in their fine motor skills. As you do art projects with your client remember your role is not to judge the client's artwork in any manner, including psychoanalyzing it. Instead, encourage and coach your client's efforts by helping them understand when they have completed the target goal of the exercise. Discussing your client's artwork is an excellent opportunity for him or her to practice their communication and thinking skills. It also helps them practice the processes of comparison and reflection.

You do not need to understand everything your client is explaining about their art. However, you must be an active listener, allowing a safe space for your client to express their thoughts, words, and feelings without opinion. Let your client guide you to how long they want to spend discussing their artwork, by paying attention to their energy and attention level.

Creating art had quite a positive impact on Jo. She was happiest when she was painting.

Not only did drawing and painting provide a pleasant distraction from her pain and anxiety, it also gave her a much-needed sense of accomplishment. She developed quite a following for her whimsical birds and the colorful women that she created. When we got her work accepted in a local gallery, it was a great morale booster for her. People were buying her prints and greeting cards. Jo and her husband attended monthly showings at the gallery. This gave Jo a chance to meet other artists, see their work, and share a good time with them. One month she was celebrated as "artist of the month!"

Whenever Jo felt depressed, I would remind her that she was accomplishing something amazing with her non-dominant hand that most people could not do. She was painting and selling her images. Jo would usually cheer up when she looked through her portfolio of paintings. She liked her birds the best and called them "her friends." I believe that they were.

HERE ARE SOME QUESTIONS TO USE WITH YOUR CLIENT TO HELP THEM CRITIQUE THEIR ARTWORK.

- Do you think you met the goal or target of this exercise?

- How is your image the same as the original image? How is it different?

- Can you tell me something about this particular part of your drawing?

- How difficult was this exercise for you?

- What do you like about your art? Why?

- Is there something you do not like? Why?

- What would you do diffewrently if you did it again?

- Would you like to do this type of exercise again? Why or why not?

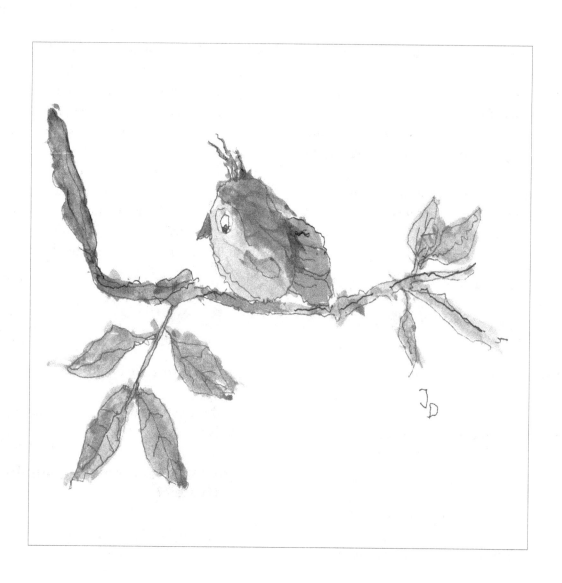

CHAPTER NINE

THE POWER OF WRITING

The moon lets the water become more of the sky. — Jo

Journal writing is an effective method for personal reflection across many disciplines. Journals are used in medical and counseling professions, businesses, educational settings and others. In the counseling profession, journal writing helps the client express feelings and process through painful emotions and events. There has been research studies done on expressive writing for healing since the early 1990s. These studies indicate that journal writing can provide many benefits, such as improvement in asthma, autoimmune disorders and pain management.

I grew up with two parents that kept journals. I learned early on about the importance of the written word. I've kept journals throughout my life and have taught workshops on reflective writing for many years. I understand the value of journal writing to record life's big events, capture memories and provide an outlet for reflection and planning. I was excited to use writing as a cognitive and creative outlet for Jo. Our journaling exercises included the use of two forms of journals: the handwritten journal and the computer journal. We began with the handwritten journal because it was immediate, accessible and simple.

Whether Jo was writing on paper or later keyboarding on the computer, her brain was working hard. She had a lot to coordinate to complete the exercise. I saw from Jo's efforts how cognitively challenging the act of forming letters and connecting them on the page can be. The ability to handwrite words legibly and write one's name became an obvious measuring stick for cognitive improvement or decline. These handwritten journal exercises were personal and emotional for Jo. Unfortunately, much of her writing was indecipherable even for her, which made her cry. Nevertheless, we both could read a few writings, and we talked about them.

It helps to have a clear intention of what type of writing you will do in the session. Will it be writing for self-awareness? Will it be creative writing such as storytelling or poetry? Knowing the intention will help you structure the lesson better. With that being said, do not be surprised if a creative writing exercise suddenly takes a turn and becomes deeply introspective or if a journal writing passage reads like a fantasy or a poem. This will happen and that is the wonder of the writing journey--it is a path of many paths.

WRITING EXERCISES

When we began writing, my goal for Jo was to write three complete sentences. It did not come easy for her and I would watch her repeatedly type the same word, sentence or phrase with maybe a slight variation. Sometimes, it took her a half an hour or longer to type three simple sentences. The process required her to press the letter key down with just the right amount of pressure so the letter appeared on the screen once instead of twenty times. She also had to remember how to spell the words she typed, all the while focusing on what she wanted to say. Not an easy feat for a stroke survivor, or anyone with aphasia.

After Jo had been writing for some time, I decided it was time to raise the cognition bar higher! Now, instead of three sentences she had to type a paragraph (six sentences) without any repetition of words or sentences. She also had to stay on topic. I usually typed the topic or prompt at the top of the page or had it written on a piece of paper by the side of the computer where she could find it. I always provided her with written directions and showed her where she could find them. It was important to me that she could locate information whenever she needed---an important step towards future independence.

EXERCISE: Free Write

Directions: Have your client write about anything they want. Let them know that there are no rules, and typos and grammar issues are not a concern. It is more important to get the thought out than worry about how it is typed or written at this point. There is no right or wrong way to do this exercise. Although to complete the exercise successfully, the client needs to focus on writing or typing for the prescribed amount of time (15 minutes or whatever the client can tolerate).

Jo and I used this exercise often. I liked it because it gave Jo creative freedom and stimulated her thinking skills. Jo worked as hard on these exercises as she would have in a gym. She not only had to coordinate her thought processes to come up with information but also retain it, remembering how to spell, while her non-dominate hand had to learn to write or type them. It was a great exerciser for brain, hand and eye coordination. These journal moments were very important therapy for Jo. They

gave her freedom to be with herself, alone and relaxed, while letting her thoughts flow freely. I know she had many more thoughts during those times than she could finger peck with one hand. Therefore, in a sense, these sessions also served as quiet, reflective moments that were very rare in her rehabilitation schedule. Jo also did not complain that much about pain when she was concentrating on her writing.

EXERCISE: Timed Writing

Let your client know that this will be a short, five-minute timed writing. Ask your client to write or type for five minutes on any topic or word of their choice. If they cannot think of anything, suggest an idea for them to use. Write the topic or word at the top of the page. Sometimes, for this activity, I presented Jo with a pile of bright little cards with inspirational words on them such as compassion, light, energy, peace, hope, etc. This is a good writing warm up exercise.

EXERCISE: Journaling to Photographs or Images

Directions: Have your client select photographs or images that appeal to them. Let them have a few moments to absorb the image. Then ask them to write in their journal a response to the following questions:

- What is happening in this image?

- What do you feel when you look at these photos?

- What do you want to say to the people, places, or things in these photos?

- Have you ever had a similar experience?

EXERCISE: Prompts

Prompts can be words, statements, questions, lyrics, poetry, etc. Prompts are everywhere around you. They simply are starting points from which your writing can take off and lead you down a direction. Here are ten simple writing prompts:

1. I am...
2. I love...
3. I know...
4. I feel...
5. I want...
6. I will...
7. I can...
8. I hope...

Directions: The client picks out a prompt they would like to write about or you can suggest one. Put the prompt in a prominent place so they can see it. Time the writing for whatever is appropriate for your client between five and 30 minutes. Client is encouraged to share their writing, but only if they want. An atmosphere of trust is important when sharing writings with others, and it can take time to build. If your client wants to share what they have written, invite them to read it aloud. Further discussion may naturally follow.

Here is an example of Jo's writing using the prompt, *What do you like?*

Observe and watch people. See what I can learn from them.
Like to be outside in good weather.
Enjoy nature, and birds.
See people who are happy and doing things with their family and children.
More free time.
See my children.
Read. I love to read about what people are doing.
Like to play piano.
Like to write about children and myself.
Write books, children's books and stories.
Like to do art.

More Writing Prompts:

1. If you could travel anywhere in the world where would you go? Why?
2. What would you want if you had three wishes?
3. If you knew you would not fail, what would you do?
4. The best thing in life is...
5. What gift would you like to give yourself this year?
6. What is your favorite color? How does it make you feel?

EXERCISE: Gratitude List

A simple yet uplifting exercise where the client will write in a list form what they are thankful for in their lives. A goal of ten things is a good starting place.

Here is a sample of Jo's Gratitude List:

1. Being with people.
2. Being with children.
3. Sharing with people.
4. Talking with people.
5. Going outside.
6. Enjoying what comes.
7. Reading books about other people's adventures.
8. Helping others.
9. Gardening.
10. Cooking.
11. Care of house.
12. Plays and concerts

EXERCISE: Metaphor: What Element in Nature Describes You Best?

A metaphor is a figure of speech that describes one thing as something else.

Directions: Client writes about an element in nature that they feel they are like. Examples could be: elements like rain, fire, snow, earth;

water, trees, plants flowers; clouds, stars, sun and moon; animals, birds or insects; rocks, rivers, mountains and oceans. There is no right or wrong way of completing the exercise.

Sample of Jo's metaphor writing:

> I have wings and I can fly high in the sky. I also have areas to roost upon. It has flowers and space to bring friends. It also has areas to bring food to birds that need it. I am also able to show how to bring food to friends who need it.

EXERCISE: Write a Story from a Different Point of View

There are two different points of view a person can write from: first person (oneself) using the words "I and me," and third person (other) using the words "she, her and he, him.

Previously, Jo and I had been talking about fear issues and we were trying to get to the root of them. Jo had used the words "trapped" and "lost," in our conversation. When I heard them, I knew they could be writing prompts. Jo dictated the story and I wrote as fast as I could. The words just flowed out of her and I had a hard time keeping up with her! It was great.

(Mistakes intentionally left in)

> Once upon a time, there was...
> A little girl who was trapped. She was walking with her mother and she got lost. She was in the forest. She couldn't find her way out. The little girl was excited. She tried to find her way out...her way home...but she lost her way in the forest. There were people walking in the forest. They didn't think she wanted or could take the time to be with the people. They couldn't include her in their activities. She feels lost and left out.

(Same exercise, second version)

> A young woman got lost. She lost her way along the road. There was lots of fresh air. The road was a pathway. People took the path. They were people who knew how to get around. But she didn't have time to bother herself, so she went along the path and followed the others who walked along the path. But they never involved her in their time. She found herself in a place where she could sleep and she found she could take sleep anytime she needed to. It helped her wake up refreshed so she could do more.

On the third attempt at this writing exercise, Jo switched to "I" statements and began writing about herself. This writing technique is powerful because it gives the writer an opportunity to express their thoughts and feelings from a "safe" distance. By using this technique, the writer can become more observant of their life. It is a very good exercise for exploring difficult or emotional issues.

Another way to use this exercise is to write from a completely different point of view such as the viewpoint of a tree or a bird. This is a fun exercise that encourages creativity. The following is a list of ideas for different viewpoints:

- A Christmas tree on Christmas Eve.
- A pod of whales.
- A wedding chapel in Las Vegas.
- A bird on a branch in a snowstorm.
- A clown.
- A bus driver.
- A dog when its master comes home.
- A cat on the windowsill.

EXERCISE: Finish the Sentence

This is a fun exercise that encourages creativity. Provide your client with one of the following sentence stems to finish or come up with your own ideas.

1. She opened the book and read the words...
2. Inside the gift box was a very small...
3. He did not believe in magic until...
4. The dog was digging in the ground when he found a...
5. In the garden grew the most beautiful...
6. She wrote a letter to...
7. The boy left the room to find...
8. There was a room in the old house where...
9. It was just a matter of time before they found out...
10. The wind blew so hard that it...

EXERCISE: The Unsent Letter

Have your client select someone to be the recipient of the unsent letter. They can write to anyone, living, deceased or even imaginary. They can write to different parts of themselves such as the nurturer, the doer, the unbeliever or the person they were before their stroke, etc.

This exercise is often used for writing to a loved one who has passed on or to a person that you will never see again but with whom you have unresolved issues. Be aware that this exercise might bring up some strong emotional reactions in your client depending on the depth and direction of their writing.

EXERCISE: Dialogue

This is a writing technique, well known and used by psychotherapists, to elicit a dialogue between two different parts or viewpoints of their patient. The dialogue can consist of interaction between the inner child and the adult self, the body and the mind, the past self and the future self, an illness and the self, and many other scenarios. This exercise emphasizes different viewpoints, without judgement and creates an awareness of inner struggles that might not be so obvious to the writer.

EXERCISE: Your Perfect Day

This is a straightforward exercise. Turn on some pleasant music and give your client a few moments to consider what their perfect day would look like. Encourage them to consider as many details as possible to make it come alive in their minds. Who are they with? Where do they live? What are they doing? This exercise usually takes 20 to 30 minutes.

POETRY WRITING

Poetry challenges the brain and offers us a different perspective in which to interpret the world. Researchers have found that poetry, with its rhymes, rhythms and alliterations, works like music does on our brains to elicit emotions and memories. Poetry is a good cognitive workout that can be both pleasurable and stimulating.

Jo enjoyed our poetry reading sessions; one of her favorite authors that we read was Robert Frost. Interestingly, I found that Jo could repeat back a poetic phrase much better than she could ordinary prose. She was also finding connections between the poems we read and the world around her. For example, when we read "The Road Not Taken" by Robert Frost, she said that she too "was on the path few take."

We began our poetry sessions with haiku, a traditional form of Japanese poetry composed of 17 syllables in three lines that usually do not rhyme. The most common themes are nature, a profound moment, something of beauty, or universal truth. The first and last lines of a Haiku have five syllables, and the middle line has seven syllables. The syllable is the division of sound you hear in a word. Example, the word *water* has two syllables.

We read haiku from masters Matsuo Basho and Natsume Soseki for inspiration. The structure of haiku is simple, but the imagery and meaning can be very profound. Here are two haiku poems Jo wrote. Although, they do not follow the haiku formula exactly, they are wonderful little expressions.

> Light from above
> Jumping up and down on water
> Dancing diamonds.

> It is slow
> It is white
> It follows the light.

EXERCISE: Haiku

Directions: Select a subject. If the focus is nature, it might be trees, leaves, stars, clouds, animals, rivers, birds, ocean, fish, flowers, etc.

Brainstorm words that describe the subject in your haiku. Here are some descriptive words you could consider when writing about autumn leaves: rusted, crunchy, fragrant, spicy, brittle, glowing, or slender. Think of your senses as you collect words. How does the subject you are writing about look, smell, feel, taste and sound? This is a good exercise I used with Jo to practice word retrieval. It is fun and simple and she enjoyed it very much.

Haiku sample form:

> Line One: _____
> Line Two: _____
> Line Three: _____

EXERCISE: Free Form Poetry

Free form poetry does not have any consistent meter, rhyme or any other musical pattern or restrictions. It often tends to follow the rhythm of natural speech. It is a very freeing and fun way to write poems. If your client enjoys writing free form poetry look for books and online sites that provide samples and inspiration.

Here are four short examples of free form poetry written by Jo:

> It's warm outside, happy little birds.
> Keep your eye on the day
> Keep your bad thoughts away
> Listen to the happy birds sing.

> The moon lets the water become more of the sky.
> You can climb a mountain to see the light
> You can see the sky become larger.
> The closer you get to it... the larger it becomes.
> Stars get you above the clouds.
> Walk up the clouds to the stars.

> When you learn, your way out it is better.
> You find someone to teach you the way.
> Sometimes you are okay.

COMPUTER KEYBOARDING AS A COGNITIVE EXERCISE

You can show your client how to use the computer keyboard by helping them with navigating the keys, handling the mouse, opening applications, and using the internet. Help them as much or as little as needed. There are wonderful online brain games websites, stroke websites and support groups, and other informative sites to help them make connections and learn about the world.

I introduced keyboarding after we began our journaling activities so that Jo could express her thoughts and feelings quicker and hopefully read her typed words better. The computer had its advantages such as a large, well-lit screen, variable font sizes, ability to correct, and ability to save writings. It also provided some extra cognitive challenges. I was very excited about how the computer, with its keyboard, mouse, letter and functions keys, etc., would serve as a teaching tool.

Let us begin by taking a moment to break down the major steps involved to operate a word processing program on a laptop commuter. I think many of us take these steps for granted and do not realize immense challenge it is for those who are cognitively and/or physically challenged. Not all these steps will be applicable in all situations.

1. Transporting oneself to the computer.
2. Opening the laptop cover.
3. Turning on the computer or laptop.
4. Entering a password, if applicable.
5. Opening up desired programs.
6. Know how to operate the mouse or finger pad.
7. Navigating the keyboard and understanding the backspace, delete, tab, shift, and other commonly used keys.
8. Knowing how to eliminate a dialogue box when it pops up.
9. Select a word processing program to use.
10. Know how to operate the program, such as correcting errors, page down, page up, etc.
11. Know how to open, save, retrieve and close a document.
12. Know how to exit the program.
13. Know how to shut down computer.
14. Leaving the computer station.

Using only your non-dominate hand to type on a computer keyboard is difficult. But, consider doing that along with having hand spasms, vision issues, and word retrieval and concentration difficulties. Those are the challenges Jo faced. I had to offer a significant amount of assistance to her when we started out on the computer. I would turn on the computer, open the word program to a blank document, set the font style and font size and turn on the caps. In addition, I covered the control, shift, delete and alt keys with tape so that she could steer clear from accidently hitting them. I also put bright tape on the backspace and enter keys. I purchased a set of large stick-on keyboard stickers to help her see the letters clearly. In addition, the keyboard was placed on a non-skid, elevated surface and the mouse was repositioned for her left hand. Then she was ready to go!

HOW TO ASSESS WRITING EXERCISES

- How many sentences were completed during a 20 -30-minute writing session?

- How often did the client need cues to remember the writing topic?

- Did the client stay on track with the writing topic or veer off to something else?

- How many times did client repeat the same sentence or phrase during the session?

- How many new or novel thoughts or words was client able to express?

- How many grammatical or typing errors did client's writing contain?

- How many words did not make sense?

- Was the client able to articulate what they had written?

SCRIBING

Jo's inability to use her dominant hand to write or type and her struggle to control her fine motor skills with her non-dominant hand required me to act as her scribe on occasion. Generally, I only scribed for her when she asked me to, either because she was too tired to write or because she had more to say than she could type without exhaustion and frustration. When we wrote our short stories together, I usually typed for her to allow her time to imagine the story and its characters. Other than those times, Jo did her own typing, including emails.

Scribing is an excellent tool to use either if your client does not have the use of their hands. It will assist those that have vision problems or have another condition or situation that prevents them from writing or typing themselves. There are advantages to scribing. First, the client can express his or her thoughts in a more flowing, uninterrupted manner, without struggling to find the correct letters on the keyboard. By removing the mechanical step of actually typing on the keyboard, the client can concentrate better on what words they want to say, which is often challenging enough. It gives the non-dominant hand a much-needed rest, and it builds intimacy and trust between client and coach.

If you are going to scribe for someone, accuracy and patience is paramount. You want to write down the exact words your client said without substitution or "improving" on them, even if the language is incorrect. Make grammar and spelling corrections later, if at all. When scribing, you will need to stop periodically and show or read the transcription to the client so that they can approve of it. I would often ask Jo, Is this what you want to say? Did I understand you correctly? Do we need to make changes? I would ask her to point to the words on the screen that needed to be changed.

Many times, Jo had me retype some of her statements because either I could not fully understand her words or because once she saw them typed, she changed her mind. Jo was very adept at pointing out any typos that I made-- which made me happy because it indicated her alertness to detail.

Three examples of Jo's scribed writings with typos intentionally left in:

Example One:

THE ANGEL OF JOY

I love this little girl who
Comes inside to
Bring gifts to all
The gifts are brought to all and include the following

The peace, love, smiles, and laufture
The girls were happy
With their gifts
They were also pleased with the other gifts

And most of all they engoyed their drink of white wine
Their wine was more than tasty
The wine had a taste of its own.
Merry Christmas to all.

Example Two:

Keep your eyes open to all thoughts Listen to their thoughts. Listen how they sound. Pay attention. They all have thoughts. They're wanting to come over. They want to participate. We listen to the ideas, we give them food, comfort. We listen to their words. They want to be part of what is happening.

Example Three:

Becoming again like they were in the beginning. The birds are part of this. My friend has been free to choose his own way to live. Free to make his choice in friends. Suddenly, it isn't just the way things happen. Sometimes we have to give of ourselves. The freedom to come and go whenever they want.

As a cognitive coach, you will not be using journal writing therapeutically. Naturally, there might be sensitive issues that surface because most all journal writing is revealing when written openly and honestly. Do not dwell on or overly explore these issues unless you are a licensed therapist equipped with coping skills to offer your client. As a coach, you are there as a silent witness providing a safe place for your clients to express themselves through the act of writing.

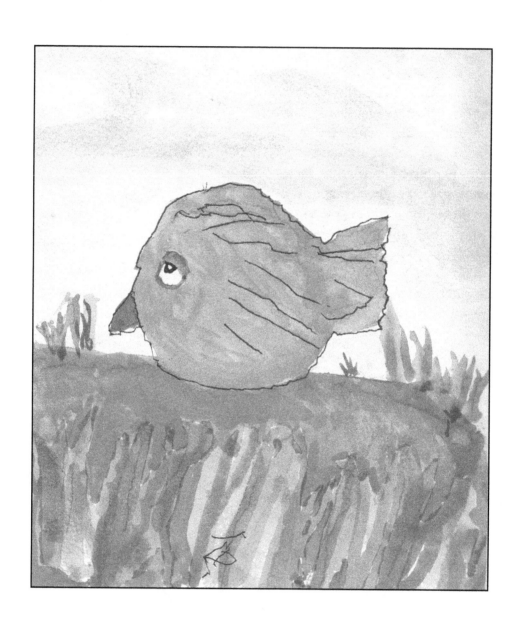

CHAPTER TEN

THE HEALING POWER OF STORYTELLING

Once Upon a Time...

Everybody loves a good story. Stories help us make sense of our world while stimulating our imagination. Stories have helped people recover from post-traumatic stress syndrome, personal loss, physical illness, traumatic brain injuries, and even high blood pressure! I decided to add the story-writing component to the curriculum to improve Jo's attention, memory, visual processing, language, and reasoning skills.

Stories that are read or listened to demand many cognitive skills. I knew Jo would have to be able to pay attention and concentrate on the story. Then she would have to organize the incoming information (audio or visual) and make sense of the story. Finally, she would have to remember the information as she attempted to use language skills to answer questions or make comments on it. Over the years, Jo showed continued improvement in the story writing part of the program. Sometimes her ability to retrieve memories and find the correct words to describe them was very good, other times, she had difficulty. It depended on how she was feeling emotionally and physically.

I found that the storytelling component of the program was a powerful one, not only because of the cognitive and communication challenges it presented but also because it helped Jo strengthen her interpersonal skills (self-understanding). It was a fun tool to help her build vocabulary and work on speech. It allowed her the opportunity to articulate her thoughts. This is important since too often stroke leaves people feeling a loss of identity and frustrated. The act of sharing a personal story can also encourage trust and intimacy between two people.

I decided to explore several different approaches to storytelling. Since Jo was not able to type or write the story with her non-dominant hand without struggling with motor ability, we agreed that she would dictate the story to me, and I would scribe it for her. There were several initial challenges involved in this activity. First, she had to be able to organize her thoughts into a narrative and find the appropriate words. Second, she had to remember her thoughts and words. Third, Jo had to be able to articulate her words so that I could understand them. Lastly, she had to be able to recall her story from day to day. This activity provided her with many cognitive challenges as well as enjoyment. Her brain was working hard, but she was having a great time! I believe we get the best results when learning is fun and engaging.

Here are several different types of story formats that I used with Jo. Although some stories appear to use the same technique, there are subtle differences that bring about a different outcome. Here is an example of two of our short bird stories that we wrote together.

FIONA

Fiona is a young female bird. She is not full grown yet. She has a long tail feather and long wavy dark orange feathers on her head. Her tail feathers and her head feathers are both still growing. She is very pretty with her orange beak, big blue eyes, bright yellow body and green wings. Fiona likes to pretend she is grown up. She fluffs up her feathers to look bigger than she is. She likes to dance a lot. She likes to go to places where the others are. She is quite the dancer and likes to jump around on her tiptoes and flutter her wings. Fiona likes to eat fresh food. She particularly likes green food, like vegetables and fruit. Her favorite food is grapes.

RUSSELL

Russell has many friends and likes to talk and share about happiness throughout the day. Russell is a really fun bird. We spend a lot of time together and I really like him a lot. Russell talks and visits with friends about what they are doing each day and what they like to do. They visit each other every day for afternoon snacks and to share conversation. Russell and his friends like to eat peanut butter and sunflower seed sandwiches, oranges, strawberries, and all kinds of nut and seed breads. They enjoy watermelon wine and blackberry juice with their food. Randall loves to eat best of all, and it is great fun to him.

Some of Russell's friends play musical instruments, and all his friends love to sing. Russell likes to try many different things. He is also very good at listening to his friends. He gives reliable advice.

He listens to others, and they listen to him. He is smart, trustworthy, and a good thinker. He likes to think a lot. Russell is not young, not old, but in the middle. He runs a lot and likes to be active. Sometimes he runs to different territories. He dislikes people who talk a lot. It is hard to meet others like him. Russell enjoys being alone and does not like to be crowded. He likes to be free to talk, free to listen and free to move about.

EXERCISE: Partner Stories

This is an exercise where I would start Jo with a sentence from which she would add a sentence to support or embellish the first sentence. The idea was to keep a story going like a volleyball game and create a story that made sense. However, that does not always have to be the criteria. Sometimes, just the practice of retrieving words and creating complete sentences is enough, especially in the beginning.

Here is an example of a partner Story:

Me: Once upon a time, there was a fairy godmother and she….
Jo: She liked to help people.
Me The fairy godmother decided to help two little girls so she…
Jo: Gave each of them a special gift.
Me: One gift was a magic mirror. The other gift was….
Jo: A sparkly black dress.

EXERCISE: Third-Person Stories

This exercise uses the words: "he or she" and "his and her" rather than the first-person voice of "I and me." This activity helps the client express something but does not quite know how to do it. As mentioned in the previous chapter, third-person voice automatically offers a safe sense of detachment. The storyteller becomes an observer. Often, they are not aware at the beginning of the story that they are writing about themselves or issues that concern them. This revelation usually comes later or sometimes not at all. Sensitive issues, like emotional trauma, appear disguised as belonging to someone else, usually the main character of the story.

The interpretation of the story is not the job of the family member or coach, only the one telling the story and ONLY if they choose to talk about it. The point of these stories is to provide a safe outlet for the storyteller to express their thoughts and feelings.

Here is an example of a third person story that Jo and I did:

Me: Once upon a time, there was a young woman…
Jo: A young woman who got lost. She lost her way along the road. There was lots of fresh air. She saw a lot of road but no people. The road was a pathway. People took the path.
Me: Who were these people?
Jo: They were people who knew how to get around. But she did not have time to bother herself, so she went along the path and followed the others who walked the path. But they never involved her in their time.
Me: What did she do?
Jo: She walked off the path and found herself in a place she could sleep and she found she could take sleep anytime she needed to. Sleep helped her wake up refreshed so she could do more.

It was obvious that the theme of her story was about being "lost" and feeling left out. I decided to help her explore these feelings by asking some pointed questions.

Me: What does "being lost" mean to you?
Jo: You can't find yourself a way out.
Me: What does being trapped mean to you?

Jo: Not being able to be yourself and do what you want to do or think or say.
Me: What are the problems the young woman has?

It was at this point in the conversation that Jo's answers took on the first-person voice and she responded with "I," instead of, "she or her". This type of storytelling served its purpose very well. It gave Jo the ability to tap into her feelings while being incognito and putting distance between herself and the main character. After she started to answer some specific question, she switched into the first-person voice. Obviously, she had felt safe enough to do this integration of voices.

How can this activity help your loved one or client? This third-person voice technique allows one to feel safe accessing their emotions and then expressing them through the guise of a third party. By integrating these emotions into their awareness, they realize that these emotions are a real part of themselves, and it is okay to talk about them. Asking your client specific questions about certain topics of the story might help guide them into finding their solutions or revelations about their own situation. Of course, this third person voice does not always change into a first-person voice. That is perfectly okay, it does not have to get to that place. Always allow your client to tell the story in his or her own way.

EXERCISE: Personal Stories

These stories are about personal experiences and memories. These stories stimulate memory and help the stroke survivor gain personal insight. These stories usually start with a prompt. Here is an example of a personal story.

Me: What is your favorite creature?
Jo: Birds have always given me joy. They are like real people to me, each with different personalities. I have always enjoyed birds since I could remember. When I was

little, we had a small bird that learned to say "hello and goodbye" and many other words. My brother, sister and I would take turns talking to him and teaching him what to say.

Another example:

Me: What do remember about Christmas growing up?
Jo: Christmas means being all together. I remember Christmases past with my father, mother, sister and my brother. On Christmas Eve afternoon my sister and brother helped my mother prepare dinner. Some of the food our mother made was pasta and fresh bread. We also had a variety of fish, which was soaked overnight. It was neat having our neighbors come over and join us in the cooking and eating. Food was prepared and then we ate it in the evening. My mother made fresh and good food.

STORY WRITING EXERCISES

EXERCISE: Writing Stories From Prompts

Have your client write a paragraph or two using one of the following prompts.

1. If you could do something you have never done before, what would it be? Why would you do it?

2. What do you consider to be your greatest accomplishment?

3. Describe someone you admire and explain why.

4. Talk about a time in your life when you struggled with choice. How did your choice turn out?

5. Did you ever get lost in a strange town?

6. Did you ever win or lose a contest? What happened?

7. Were you ever in a hospital? What was that like?

8. What is the funniest thing that ever happened to you?

9. What is the most beautiful thing in nature to you?

10. What is the most exciting thing you ever experienced?

11. Describe your favorite vacation.

12. Did you ever dress up for a fancy occasion? What did you wear? Where did you go?

13. Did you ever have a favorite pet? What was it? What was its name? What did you do with your pet?

14. What did you like and dislike about school or college? What were your favorite subjects in school?

15. What do you like or dislike about your job?

16. If you could go on a trip, where would you like to go?

17. What would happen if animals could talk? What are some of the questions you would like to ask animals?

18. What would happen if you could become invisible whenever you wanted to? What are some of the things you could do that you cannot do now?

19. If you had to describe yourself as a color, what color would you choose? Why?

20. What is the best advice you ever received?

21. What is your favorite holiday? What makes this holiday special?

22. If you could have been someone in history, who would you have been?

23. If you could only take three people with you on a trip around the world, who would you take and why?

24. If you could give any gift in the world, what would you give and to whom?

25. If you could live anywhere in the world, where would it be?

EXERCISE: Story Builders

The goal of this exercise is to answer each of the questions: who, what, where, when and why?

Try using the following prompts or invent your own.

1. It was an old photograph of…

2. The tree began to speak…

3. It was an unusual map that led to…

4. Something moved inside the dark cave…

5. He opened up the box and out popped…

6. The bus ended up in an unknown part of town…

7. When staring out the window I saw…

8. My friends made plans to do something fun…

9. From the first moment, I saw it…

10. The last time I saw her she was…

EXERCISE: Writing Stories from Images

Select an image that is inspiring, shows action or has vivid scenes. These images can be real or make believe.

Ask your client the following questions about the image:

1. What do you think is happening in this picture?

2. What is that person thinking?

3. What do you think that person will do next?

4. If you were that person, what would you do?

5. Does this image remind you of someone you know? Maybe yourself?

EXERCISE: Creating Stories with Found Words

Words are in a variety of places: newspapers, magazines, online, cards, advertisements and can serve as generators of stories.

Directions:

1. Cut out printed words and sentences from magazines, books or newspapers.

2. Have client arrange the words or sentences to create a mini story.

3. Glue the words and sentences to a firm background.

4. Read the finished story.

Tip: If your client has difficulty handling a scissors, let them do the selecting of the images and found words and you cut them out. Variation: You can also use magnetic poetry words for this exercise.

EXERCISE: The 26 Sentence Story

Directions:

1. Begin the first sentence with the letter "A."

2. Start the next sentence and all following sentences with the next letter of the alphabet.

3. Continue to the end of the alphabet. Have fun reading the story aloud.

BENEFITS OF READING

Because reading is a full brain activity, it is also a wonderful cognitive activity. The reader is continually shifting from letter recognition to word recognition to word meaning and finally word production. Long-term memory is stimulated as the reader relates what they are currently reading to information stored previously in their brain. Also, research has shown that these "reading" areas of the brain, in particular the left temporal cortex, remain "lit up" even after the reading session is concluded.

Another effect of reading on the brain is that it triggers a phenomenon known as "grounded cognition" which means that just thinking about dancing can activate the same neurons associated with the physical act of dancing, similar to what occurs in visualization activities. This would lead one to assume that reading encourages overall brain communication and neuroplasticity. With repeated practice, reading aloud can help with articulation, intonation, breathing and speaking rhythms. Reading aloud has the advantage of working the muscles that produce speech. It is also an opportunity to recognize how one's voice sounds, which may encourage one to speak more clearly. Your client can hear where their reading was monotone or if they varied their speech patterns. You can record your client while they read and play it back for them to hear. Observe their reading speed and pronunciation of words

Like any of the activities and exercises in this book, you want to work with your client's ability level. This might mean doing reading comprehension exercises from grade books. This is the place I started with Jo to test her reading comprehension and retention abilities. These gradebooks are useful because the reading material is usually one to three short paragraphs on simple subject matter. There are questions to answer after reading the paragraph. Most reading comprehension activities will require that the reader put the main points of the paragraph in sequential order.

Here is an example:

Sally woke up and saw that it was raining. She put on her raincoat and took her umbrella with her. Sally walked to the store. At the store, Sally bought some apples and oranges. Sally took a taxi home because it was raining hard. Sally cut up an apple and ate it with an orange.

Please put the sentences in the order that they occurred in the story:
___Sally took a taxi because it was raining hard.
___Sally cut up an apple.
___At the store, Sally bought some apples and oranges.
___She put on her raincoat and took her umbrella.

You can always find an interesting paragraph or two on a subject that might interest your client and develop your own questions. The best questions to ask are the news reporter's questions of **who, what, where, when, why**

and how. You can cut out newspaper or magazine articles and highlight paragraphs you want your client to read, or if vision is a difficulty, you can re-type the article in a larger font for them to read. Of course, if you have access to a computer, there are many opportunities to find material to read.

EXERCISE: Reading for Retention

Directions:

1. Ask your client what type of stories they like.

2. Select a story that is appropriate for your client's level of comprehension and attention span.

3. Read the story aloud in a quiet space, free of distractions.

4. Pause several times to recap the story.

5. After finishing the story, ask your client questions about the story.

The following questions are some ideas to help stimulate recall and conversation. Feel free to come up with your own.

1. What is the story about?

2. Who is the main character?

3. What is happening to the main character?

4. What does the main character want?

5. What challenges or problems does the main character face?

6. How does the main character solve the problem/s?

7. What would you have done if you were the main character?

8. What personality traits does the main character possess?

9. What questions would you like to ask the main character?

10. What are the most important events of the story?

11. How do you think the story will end?

12. What do you think the most important thing is to remember about this story?

13. Can you retell the important events of the story from beginning to end in your own words?

14. What was your favorite part of the story?

15. Did you like the story? Why?

16. What would you change about the story if you could?

Here is an interesting experiment to try. First, have your client read silently to themselves. After your client finishes reading, ask them several questions about what they read. How many questions could they answer correctly? Next, have them read the same material aloud. Do you notice any difference in retention or ability to answer the same questions? Lastly, you can test their auditory and attention skills by reading the material to them while they listen. Follow up with the same list of questions. What, if any differences do you notice? What method seems to be the most useful?

Not too easy--not too hard! If your client consistently answers the questions correctly and quickly, increase the complexity of the reading material. Remember--you want to provide challenging (just within reach) exercises, not overwhelmingly hard ones. You want your client to succeed and as they do, congratulate them on their achievements and move up to the next level.

EXERCISE: Reading the News

Look at a newspaper or go to the USA online news site. Select one of the top stories. Read the story aloud with your client, (you can take turns reading aloud). Then, discuss the following questions:

1. What is the story about?

2. Where is it from? What happened?

3. When did this happen? How?

4. Why did this happen?

5. What is your opinion on this event?

Here is a link to all the newspapers in the United States. http://www.usnpl.com

Stories On Tape

I am a great believer in "stories on tape or CD." I would encourage the use of them each day if possible. Audio stories help a person "see" images in their mind that the story words evoke. They also help strengthen auditory processing skills. With recorded stories, there are only words and nothing else, except perhaps some background music. A person has to work harder to visualize the unfolding events of the story because there is no added stimulation or distractions such as colors, faces, movement, etc., which happens when a person watches a movie or television show.

Movies and television also serve as cognitive stimulation, especially if subtitles are running during the show. In the beginning when I introduced audio stories, I selected children's stories. I chose them for two reasons, first, Jo had an interest in writing children's stories and second, because they usually have simpler story plots and easier to follow. A great one to listen to is the *Narnia Chronicles* and other award-winning children's stories. Jo enjoyed them immensely and when we completed them, she said, "Now, that's a real story!"

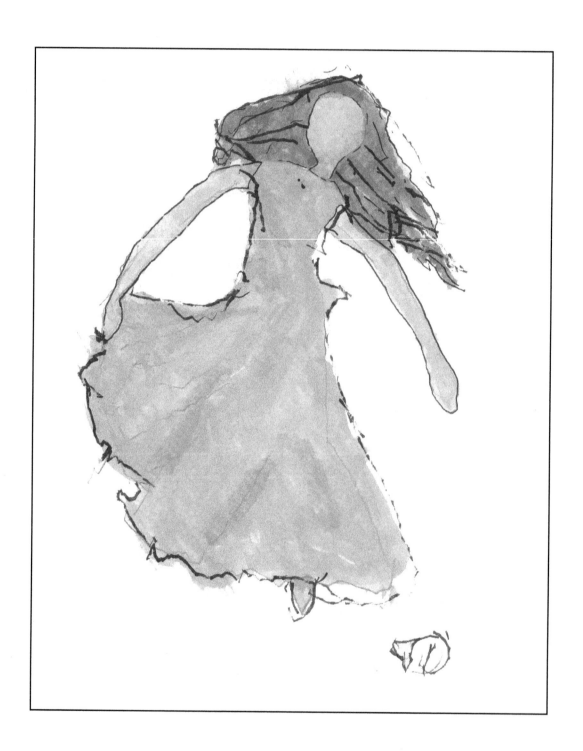

CHAPTER ELEVEN

THE BRAIN ON MUSIC

When words fail, music speaks. — SHAKESPEARE

This music chapter was the hardest for me to write because I do not have years of experience playing an instrument or reading music. I always used to say, that "I wasn't musical," until I uttered those words to a guest speaker at my graduate school. He sternly, but kindly, admonished me by saying that "everyone is musical." That guest speaker was Ellis Marsalis, legendary jazz pianist. Ever since that day, I tried to follow his advice about letting more music into my life and finding the musicality within me.

Deciding to use music as a cognitive tool provided me an opportunity to explore this world further. I began to understand that music is innate to our species, and that talent varies from person to person and can be influenced by one's environment and other factors. I also realized that even though one does not play or read music, it doesn't mean that they can't appreciate or be involved with music and enjoy its benefits.

I am thankful that I grew up in a home where my father played musicals, operas, classics and big band tunes on the weekends. It taught me to appreciate the many styles of music. Jo's musical memory included songs from the 40s, 50s, 60s. When it came to just listening to music together, we had a wide range to choose from. It was fun to sing songs from the 50s and 60s that had catchy "hooks." Jo enjoyed Duke Ellington, Benny Goodman and Glen Miller and we would watch their performances on You-Tube. We also watched operas and musicals like *Singing in the Rain, The Sound of Music,* and more. Musicals are wonderful because they have lyrics, music, color, dance and storytelling all rolled up into a visual performance. Musicals appeal to both visual and auditory learners.

Jo had been familiar with playing the piano. She had one in her home and had played it occasionally before her stroke. I was hoping that by relearning the piano keys and notes that her musical memory would resurface. I wondered if she would instinctively remember the names of the keys and their location on the keyboard. Would she suddenly recall a song that she had once played before? Would her muscle memory come into action? I was curious to find out. The more I learned about the positive effects that music had on the brain, the more excited I was to try it.

Current research has shown music to be a powerful mood enhancer and brain stimulator. Music activates both the left and right hemispheres of the brain and enables our brain to process information better and access our memories. Neuroscience is exploring music's effects on memory and learning. They have made some fantastic discoveries and are still learning more about music's impact on the brain.

Benefits of Playing an Instrument:

- Improves attention and memory.
- Improves eye and hand coordination.
- Encourages the ability to memorize sounds and patterns.
- Enhances auditory or listening skills.
- Encourages the recognition of harmonic patterns.
- Encourages active interpretation.
- Activates several regions throughout the brain.
- Increases the production of neurotransmitters like norepinephrine and melatonin.
- Stimulates memories.
- Lowers blood pressure.
- Reduces anxiety.
- Improves alertness.
- Encourages sociability.
- Improves fine motor skills.

What the researchers say:

According to Oliver Sacks, MD, Neurologist, and professor at Columbia University,

"It has been substantiated only in the last year or two that music therapy can help restore the loss of expressive language in patients with aphasia following brain injury from stroke. Beyond improving movement and speech, Sack says, Music can trigger the release of mood-altering brain chemicals and once-lost memories and emotions." [1]

Aniruddh D. Patel, Ph.D., Senior Fellow in Theoretical Neurobiology at the Neurosciences Institute states,

"Nouns and verbs are very different from tones and cords and harmony, but the parts of the brain that process them overlap." Patel also believes that music doesn't appeal to a few areas of the brain, but for large proportions of both hemispheres." [2]

Gottfried Schlaug, MD, - Neurologist, at Harvard Medical School states:

"Music appears to activate areas on the right side of the brain, suggesting that these areas pick up the slack for the damaged left side." [3]

Teppo Sarkarno, researcher at the University of Helsinki and the Helsinki Brain institute, found that stroke survivors who listened to music for a few hours a day significantly improved their recovery rate. This study was done with 54 patients who showed improvement in verbal memory, focused attention, and improved mood after two months. Sarkarnmo suggests that music should be a daily part of rehabilitation because it is targeted, easy-to-conduct, and inexpensive means to facilitate cognitive and emotional recovery. [4]

Jo and I always had background music playing during our sessions, except during speech practice. Mostly we listened to Mozart and Bach and other classical musicians. We usually started each morning singing "Que Sera Sera," sung by Doris Day, "My Favorite Things," sung by Julie Andrews and "Zippy Doo Dah," by James Baskett. After that, we were ready to start our work. It was fun and Jo seemed to enjoy our morning songs. Her voice was the clearest when she was singing.

ACTIVITY: Listening To Music

I suggest listening to a wide range of music styles. Music is a great way to elicit feelings, memories, and associations. You can talk to your client about what they liked or did not like after listening to a set of music. Watch your client's facial expressions and reactions as they listen to music, It should promote relaxation and pleasure.

I enjoyed reading Don Campbell's book, *The Mozart Effect*. He writes about how music affects the mind and body. It is a fascinating book, and I highly recommend it. I played Campbell's Mozart Effect CDs to Jo often, and both of us liked them. In his book, Campbell recommends doing a listening exploration of a variety of music genres and he describes the effects different music has on the listener.

ACTIVITY: Singing

Singing is an enjoyable cognitive exercise because it provides both enjoyment and learning. Singing helps to reinforce auditory discrimination, repetition, memory, and word identification. Certain songs can connect to specific memories and emotions. It is best to select music that has "hooks" or phrases that you cannot forget or get out of your mind. To get started, you can listen to popular songs from different decades.

Jo and I began with songs that were most familiar to both of us---patriotic songs, campfire songs, hymns, childhood songs, and Christmas carols. It was amazing to see her remember and sing the words to so many songs, even when she was having difficulty speaking.

ACTIVITY: Drawing to Music

Directions:

Select a musical piece. Provide crayons or markers or pens for client to use. The goal of the exercise is to express how the music makes your client feel on paper. The images or designs do not have to make any sense or logic. Free expression is the goal of this activity.

ACTIVITY: Shake Rattle and Roll to Music

Music has the power to energize every part of our bodies. We tap our feet, snap our fingers, and swing our bodies. Even if one cannot dance, they can move to music in a wheelchair or even lying in bed. Often Jo and I would wiggle away to the tunes of the 50s and 60s that she liked. It is an excellent way to start a session or to do in the middle of a session when energy is low. So do not forget to wiggle and dance!

PIANO BASICS

I found an electronic Casio keyboard at a second-hand store and immediately started to teach myself a few of the basics before introducing music into the program. The advantage of not knowing how to play the instrument put me in the "beginners" state of mind. As a result, I learned how to teach the fundamentals in the most natural way possible to someone who didn't know anything about music (me). I was learning for the first time while Jo was re-learning music. Learning to play the keyboard required me to focus and concentrate on new and unfamiliar material. There were new terms and symbols to understand. As I learned to play a simple song, I experienced myself making associations and recognizing patterns. My finger dexterity improved as well as my ability to remember new information. It provided a richly kinesthetic, auditory, and visual experience for me. Best of all, I felt like my brain was getting a workout. I knew at that moment that music would be an excellent cognitive tool for Jo.

A keyboard is an excellent instrument for beginners. It does not matter if you, as a coach, have any musical background. Music is such a powerful cognitive tool that I encourage you to incorporate music activities with your client or loved one. The following information is what I learned teaching the music part of our program. The activities show the progress that Jo made. If your client advances quickly or is a former musician, I recommend that you encourage them to continue to more challenging exercises.

MUSIC READING BASICS

Measures

Music is written out as notes on a staff. It consists of five lines with four spaces between them. The vertical lines on the staff separate the measures. Measures divide and organize music. The time signature determines how many beats can be in a measure. The thick double bars mark the beginning and ends of a piece of music.

Notes

The musical alphabet is, in ascending order by pitch, A, B, C, D, E, F, and G. After G, the cycle repeats going back to A. Each line and space on the staff represents a different pitch. The lower on the staff, the lower the pitch of the note. The symbol for notes is small ovals on the staff.

Notes are written on the lines or in the spaces between the lines. "EVERY GOOD BOY DOES FINE" are the words associated with the notes that **sit** on the treble clef staff lines.

The lowest note on the bottom line is E, and the note ascends to F. The notes that are **in** the spaces are F, A, C, and E. They spell out the word FACE, which is an easy way to remember these notes. F is the note in the lower space, and E is the note in the highest space. Each successive space and line is the next letter in the musical alphabet. The keyboard notes follow this pattern.

There are whole notes, half notes, quarter notes, eighth notes, and sixteenth notes. For simplicity, I chose music with a time signature of four beats represented by the whole note held for four counts. Most of the music we played used whole notes and quarter notes for ease of understanding for both Jo and myself!

A whole note is played for the full duration of the time signature. Hold down key for four counts. The half note is half the duration. Hold down key for two counts. The quarter note is half the duration of a half note or one count.

The Piano Keyboard

There are 36 black keys and 52 white keys on the keyboard for a total of 88 keys on the piano. The black ones are raised and are set farther back than the white ones. Each key on the keyboard represents a musical note. The sets of black keys are divided into sets of two and sets of three. The sets of three black keys are called "forks" and the sets of two black keys are called "chopsticks."

This is a beneficial tip so that you can always find the "C" and "F" notes. To the left of the set of two black keys is the key of "C" and to the left of the three black keys is the key of "F." This stays the same up and down the keyboard. So, you can remember because "forks" begin with "F" and "chopsticks" begin with "C." A sharp is the name for a black key to the right of (or higher than) a white key. A flat is the name for the black key to the left of (or lower than) a white key. Middle "C" is found in the middle of the keyboard. This image shows the musical notes on the keyboard starting with middle "C" shown. As you will see, the musical scale repeats itself.

Fingering

The fingers on both hands are numbered the same. Starting with the thumb (1), the pointer finger (2), the index finger, (3), the ring finger (4), and the pinkie (5). The finger positions are the same for both hands. These positions are used to play chords. The major chords are played with fingers: one, three, and five.

KEYBOARD ACTIVITIES

Even if your client does not advance to learning songs, the keyboard is still a tremendous cognitive activity to exercise motor skills and memory. Merely having your client practice going up and down the scale smoothly with their index finger will strengthen eye and hand coordination. If they can name the note they are hitting as they travel up and down the keyboard, it will help them improve their memory and association skills.

Before beginning a session, it is a good idea to do some hand stretches.

- Stretch out the fingers as far as they can go and bring them back to normal position. Do not go past the point of comfort. Do about ten stretches.

- Then take each finger and bring it down and up as if you are tapping. Do ten times.

- Then put fingertips on hard surface and tap each finger from thumb to pinkie and back again, as rapidly and smoothly as possible. Do ten times.

ACTIVITY: Introduction to The Piano Keys

Goal: To encourage finger dexterity, wrist control, and to learn the names of the keys on the keyboard.

Directions:

1. Be sure that the fingers are not flat or weighty against the keys. The ideal position is to have the fingers slightly curled as if holding a tennis ball. Elevate the wrists slightly.

2. Point out the difference between the black and white keys, explaining that the sets of two black keys will help in locating "C" and "F" keys.

3. Start with the C key and name off the keys: C, D, E, F, G, A, B, C, D, E, F, G, A, B, C.

4. Have your client name the keys as they go up the keyboard. Do the same going down the keyboard.

5. Variation: Ask your client to hit all the "C" keys. T then hit all the "A" keys, then the "F" keys. Be sure to alternate the keys to be sure they know where the keys are. Go up and down the keyboard.

6. Variation: Write a list of note strings. You can place them on a long strip of paper and place near the keyboard above the keys. Have your client read and play them in order. Example: GB-CACDEFDAGFC, etc.

ACTIVITY: Learning the Notes on a Staff or Measure (Advanced)

Goal: Encourage new learning and memory.

Directions:

1. Explain where the notes are on the staff. Let your client know they can use the memory cue "EVERY GOOD BOY DOES FINE AND FACE," to help them recall the notes. Practice going over the notes and their placement before moving on to the next step.

2. Create your own musical flash cards by drawing five lines on blank index cards and then putting in circles on the lines and spaces to show individual notes. Example: This is the "B" note. Write the note on the back of the card. Ask your client, "*What note is this*?" Do this for all the notes. Practice the cards with your client. This is the foundation of reading music.

ACTIVITY: Learning Songs

You can find on the internet many easy beginner songs that you can download. Some good sources are children's songs because they have a simple note pattern and because their melodies are familiar. It helps to have familiar songs because your client may know the tune, and it will help them learn the rhythm easier as they play. Some easy songs include: "Twinkle, Twinkle Little Star," "Itsy Bitsy Spider," "Old Macdonald," "Amazing Grace," "When the Saints Come Marching In," "Row, Row Your

Boat," Yankee Doodle Dandy, London Bridge, and more. When introducing a song, write the letters of the notes under the words, unless your client can read music.

Goal: Encourage memory, eye-hand coordination, finger dexterity

Directions:

Easy: Have the letters and notes in front of your client until they can play the song very well.

Hard: Remove the letters and note cues and have your client begin to play the song by memory.

As you look for new songs that your client can learn, find songs with the note letter written below the notes. Naturally, the letter cues are the easiest to learn. As long as your client continues to need the letter cues, write them in. If your client can read music, you can skip this step. Until that time, the cues are very helpful, and the notes will reinforce the skill of reading music. Again, work within your client's abilities. Also, be sure to work with songs that are short, easy to remember, and hopefully familiar.

Before proceeding to the next new song, be sure the current song is understood and can be played entirely with a few errors as possible. Work towards having your client self-correct their mistakes before you point them out. Increase the cognitive challenge by having the client sing along to the music they are playing. Eventually, encourage your client to play the song by memory.

ACTIVITY: Learning Chords

Learning chords is a great way to improve finger ability, memory, and association skills.

Chords: C MAJOR, F MAJOR, G MAJOR are the most commonly used chords, and they are the ones we will be focusing on in these lessons. You can find many beginner piano lessons online that provide excellent information. They include diagrams, music sheets, and videos. If your client advances quickly or is a musician, you may want to look for more challenging exercises. As a beginner myself, I found these exercises a great place to start. Finger placements for both hands are given.

C Major Chord

• **Right Hand** placement for C MAJOR Chord: The C major chord is played by placing the fingers 1, 3, and 5 on the respective keys (for right hand) as follows: Thumb (1) on key "C", middle finger (3) on key "E" and pinkie finger (5) on key "G."

• **Left-Hand** Placement for C MAJOR CHORD: If your client does not have use of their right hand and are using their left hand to play the piano, the placement will change. Then the finger placement is Pinkie (5) on key "C," middle finger (3) on key "E" and thumb (1) on key "G."

F Major Chord

• **Right Hand** placement for F MAJOR Chord: the F major chord is played by placing the fingers 1, 3, and 5 on the respective keys (for right hand) as follows: Thumb (1) on key "F", middle finger (3) on key "A" and pinkie finger (5) on key "C."

• **Left-Hand** placement for Playing F MAJOR Chord: the finger placement is: Pinkie (5) on key "F," middle finger (3) on key "A" and thumb (1) on key "C."

G Major Chord

• **Right Hand** placement for Playing G MAJOR Chord: the G major chord is played by placing the fingers 1, 3, and 5 on the respective keys (for right hand) as follows:

Thumb (1) on key "G", middle finger (3) on key "B" and pinkie finger (5) on key "D."

- **Left-Hand** placement for Playing G MAJOR CHORD - The finger placement is: Pinkie (5) on key "G," middle finger (3) on key "B" and thumb (1) on key.

ACTIVITY: Playing Three Finger Chords

Goal: Encourage memory and finger dexterity.

Directions:

1. Introduce the finger placement for middle "C" major chord, as shown above in the "basics" section. Have your client practice the chord several times in a row. Point out that they do not have to lift their fingers very far from the keys before bringing them down again on the keys. It is okay for them to arch their fingers resting on the keys if they can do so without making a sound. It is hard and requires improved motor skills.

2. Move up and down the keyboard hitting all the "C" chords.

3. Next, practice notes within the chord by striking a key with fingers, 5, 3, 1 for left hand or 1, 3, 5 for right hand. Example: with the hand position on the chord, strike the C, E, and G keys individually from pinkie to thumb and backward from thumb to pinkie. Again, the motion should be smooth and even sound. Try this activity up and down the keyboard.

4. Practice alternating steps #3 and #2. This will increase finger flexibility, along with recognizing the chord.

ACTIVITY: "F" Chord (Three fingers)

Goal: Encourage memory, new learning, and finger dexterity, visual and audio processing

Directions:

1. Introduce the finger placement for the "F" chord as shown above in the "basics" section and follow all the same steps for this chord as you did for the "C" chord.

2. Practice alternating between the "F" and "C" chords. Hold down each chord for the count of four beats. Like this: C, 2, 3, 4, F, 2, 3, 4, C, 2, 3, 4, F, 2, 3, 4, and so on.

ACTIVITY: "G" Chord (Three fingers)

Goal: Encourage memory, new learning, and finger dexterity, visual and audio processing

Directions:

1. Introduce the finger placement for the "G" chord as shown above, and follow the same steps for this chord as you did for the other two chords.

2. Practice alternating between the "F" and "C" and "G" chords. Count like this: C, 2, 3, 4, F, 2, 3, 4, G, 2, 3, 4, C, 2, 3, 4, F, 2, 3, 4 and so on.

COACH TIPS:

1. Put the letters of the keys on a piece of tape running the length of the piano keyboard next to the corresponding keys to aid in remembering key locations.

2. If you sense your client needs more challenge, feel free to improvise and

come up with your ideas at any point of the way! The goal of these exercises is to increase fine motor control, and eye and hand coordination skills along with memory. Keyboards offer a lot of sounds and instrument voices and are great fun.

PRACTICING PERCUSSION RHYTHMS

Rhythm is the soul of life. The whole universe revolves in rhythm. Everything and every human action revolves in rhythm.
　　　　　　　　　　—BABATUNDE OLATUNJI

Drums are one of the oldest and most basic forms of instruments, and they have been in use on every continent. The ancient cultures used the "talking" drum for communication as well as for healing and ceremonies. Indigenous shamans and healers of the world have used drums to promote physical and mental healing. Current studies have found that drumming can accelerate physical healing, emotional release, and can produce feelings of well-being. For cases involving Alzheimer's patients, autistic children, and other traumatized populations, drumming can have positive effects. These effects include the reduction of stress, fatigue, anxiety, and chronic pain by stimulating the production of endorphins and endogenous opiates that help with pain and anxiety.

Along with inducing relaxation, drumming has been shown to lower blood pressure and improve the immune system. Drumming has been found to beneficial in a wide range of physical ailments like cancer, migraines, multiple sclerosis, Parkinson's disease, stroke, paralysis, and other physical and emotional disorders.

Research Findings.

Cancer.
Expert Barry Bittman, MD, demonstrates that drumming in a group increases cancer-killing cells, which help the body combat cancer as well as other viruses. According to Dr. Bittman, "Group drumming tunes our biology, orchestrates our immunity and enables healing to begin." [5]

Neuroplasticity.
According to Michael Thaut, director of Colorado State University's Center for Biomedical Research in Music states,"-Rhythmic cues can help retrain the brain after a stroke or other neurological impairment, as with Parkinson's patients...""The more connections that can be made within the brain, the more integrated our experiences become." [6]

Stress.
Robert Lawrence Friedman states in his book, *The Healing Power of the Drum,*

It's hard to be having fun, playing and be stressed at the same time. Some of our stress is created from past or future thoughts of fear, worry, or regret, but it is very difficult to be stressed and be in the present moment. When one hits the drum, he or she is placed squarely in the here and now...(the) drum creates states of euphoria, induces light trance, promotes play, releases anger and promotes feelings of community and unity.[7]

Emotions.
Renowned neurologist Oliver Sacks states in *Musicophilia* that all humans, "can perceive music, perceive tones, timbre, pitch, intervals, melodic contours, harmony, and (perhaps most elementally) rhythm. He writes,

We integrate all of these and 'construct' music in our minds using many different parts of the brain. And to this largely unconscious structural appreciation of music is added an often intense and profound emotional reaction."

Drumming also synchronizes the frontal and lower areas of the brain, integrating nonverbal information from lower brain structures into the frontal cortex, producing "feelings of insight, understanding, integration, certainty, conviction, and truth, which surpass ordinary understandings and tend to persist long after the experience, often providing foundational insights for religious and cultural traditions, states Sacks.[8]

Percussion Instruments

Consider the physical condition of the client when choosing an instrument to play. Consider their eye-hand coordination, motor skills, flexibility, and strength. Some of these instruments are more adaptable than others for clients who have one weak side or who are in a wheelchair. Jo and I played with a small, (goblet-shaped) djembe drum and a hand-held frame drum. If drums prove to be too difficult to hold or manage, there are many types of percussion instruments to try as well, and that offer the same benefit.

I recommend claves (rhythm sticks) that come in pairs and are ideal for sharing. For stroke patients whose one hand is weaker, a clave can be put in that hand while the stronger hand taps out the rhythm. In cases of extreme disability, one rhythm stick is placed in the hand of the stroke patient, while the coach taps out rhythmic vibrations for the client to feel. Maracas are also inexpensive and can be shaken with one hand. Finger cymbals also come in pairs, and each cymbal has an elastic loop for putting over a finger. They provide good exercise for the fingers. Jo and I used shakers, clackers, a frame drum, and a small djembe drum.

The three timbre groups of hand percussion are: **wood** (woodblocks, clave, and clackers, etc.), **SHAKERS:** (maracas, rain sticks, cabasa) and **BELLS:** (cowbells, finger cymbals, chimes, triangles, and bells).

If the cost of purchasing instruments is prohibitive, try making homemade instruments, which can work adequately. Drums can be made from 5 lb. coffee cans and can fit comfortably between the legs. Make shakers from filling plastic water bottles with rice or beans. There are many ideas online for creating homemade instruments, and that is a fun activity in itself.

ACTIVITY: Playing Along To Music

It is fun to put on some music, break out the percussions and listen for the beat to match it or play along with it. Jo and I would listen to energetic rhythmic music like Brazilian or African and experiment with playing along. We also selected percussion rhythms on the Casio keyboard. Depending on the keyboard you have, there are many, many different rhythms to play along with. Jo would listen and attempt to match the beat. Often, she did better than I did! This energetic exercise is fun, especially when two people play together. This exercise promotes concentration, active listening skills, motor coordination, and a lot of laughter!

ACTIVITY: Following a Metronome

1. Purchase a metronome or go online for a free online metronome: **www.metronome.com**

2. Set the metronome to 60 beats a minute.

3. Practice taping foot or finger in unison with the metronome. Practice doing this for five minutes or as long as the client enjoys.

ACTIVITY: Foot and Finger Tapping

1. Begin by showing your client how to count and tap out a slow, steady 1-2-3-4-1-2-3-4 with their foot.

2. Then have them finger tap the same rhythm, with first their strong hand

and then their weak hand if possible. (Each number represents a tap.)

3. For a challenge, have clients tap out one rhythm with their foot and emphasize specific beats (such as 1 and 3) with their fingers.

ACTIVITY: Echoes

The coach will play a simple rhythm, and the client echoes it back. The goal is to reproduce the rhythm as accurately as possible. The client may go as slow as they need to, but the goal is to copy the coach's rhythm! If the client needs to go slower, the coach should also. It might help the client to close their eyes and listen first to the rhythm a few times before trying to play it. The coach can use any drum or percussion instrument to sound out the pattern. The client can respond with a similar or different percussion instrument. Example: coach on drum and client with maracas. The goal is to repeat the rhythm accurately.

Introduce a simple beat: 1,2,3,4, 1,2,3,4, etc. (Each number represents a strike or beat on the drum.) Have your client play this rhythm with their non-dominant hand or stronger hand at a slow and steady tempo. Experiment with increasing and decreasing the speed (faster/slower). Then see if your client can play with their weaker hand. They may not be able to reach as far or strike with as much strength with this hand, but that is okay. If the weak hand moves at all, that is good. All movement is good. Be sure they do not strain or hurt themselves. Try a variety of different percussion instruments. The coach and client do not need to have the same instrument. The goal is for the client to mimic the beat or rhythm that the coach plays.

ACTIVITY: Change the Emphasis

Play four beats and place emphasis on an individual beat, which is to strike the beat just a little stronger than the other beats.

1. Play this pattern with the emphasis on **1**, for six times. **1** 2 3 4, **1** 2 3 4.

2. Next place emphasis on **2**, so it would look like: 1 **2** 3 4. Play six times.

3. Next place emphasis on **3**, so it would look like: 1 2 **3** 4. Play six times.

4. Finally, emphasize the fourth beat and repeat six times.

5. Repeat exercise.

ACTIVITY: Playing With Both Hands

The goal is to have the movements smooth and with an even tempo. You can pick up the tempo later. Slower speeds with consistency are better than faster speeds with errors.

1. Simple: L L L R L.

2. Next: L R L R (left, right) using only the pads of the fingertips.

3. Then try L L R R L L R R, etc. This exercise is good for developing consistent control over hand movements.

4. Then try paradiddles for a real pattern challenge: L R L L R L R R L R L L R R, etc. Again, aim for consistency of strength and tempo. Play with no accents on any of the beats.

When you and your client have been able to play the above drills with accuracy, then it is time to advance to more challenges. You can find all sorts of patterns for two hands rhythms online.

ACTIVITY: Exploring the Percussion World

This activity is a pleasurable and a multifaceted one that stimulates cognition on many levels. It involves aural awareness (listening), speech (reading aloud), visual (watching videos), and processing of new information (focus) as well as memorization (answering questions).

Select a percussion instrument such as the djembe drum and explore the history of that particular drum. Learn about its origins, how the instrument is made and what its rhythms. Watch videos showing the drum being played by professionals and even videos giving lessons on that drum. You can explore the world of drums and percussion instruments and use them as a fun teaching tool! Use your imagination with this exercise.

*

I have focused on the keyboard and percussion in this chapter because that is what I used with Jo. I like the keyboard because of its ease of use and incredible cognitive challenge! Besides, the extraordinary sound effects on a keyboard are fun. Experiment and see what will work for you and your client. Hands, chopsticks, pencils, sticks of wood, spoons, etc. will all tap out a beat on a hard surface. Body rhythms are also a fun way to make sounds by merely clapping different body parts! I also introduced the harmonica to Jo because it is terrific for breath control. A singing bowl can help with wrist control. So have fun experimenting. Remember that music is a powerful mood enhancer. Find music that provides pleasure to your client.

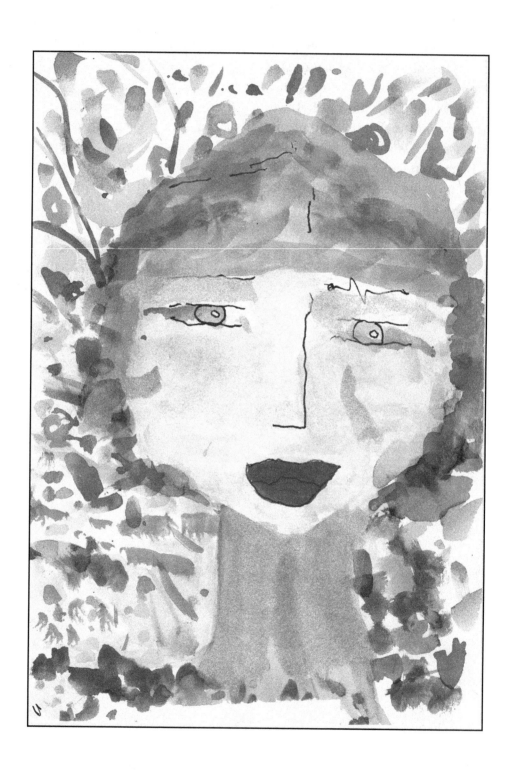

CHAPTER TWELVE

GUIDED IMAGERY

All that we are is the result of what we have thought. The mind is everything.
What we think we become. —Buddha

Distraction is a powerful tool in pain management, and many times, I needed to help Jo manage her pain by providing her with a distraction. I found that guided imagery would help her shift her focus from discomfort to relaxation and enjoyment. Usually a 20-minute imagery session provided immediate results enabling us to continue other cognitive activities.

Before starting a guided imagery session, I would be sure that Jo was in a comfortable position. That usually meant reclining her back until she was almost prone in her wheel chair. I lowered the blinds, dimmed all the lights and insured our uninterrupted privacy by putting a sign outside the door indicating a session was occurring. I used several different types of scripted imagery recordings to see which were the most effective or which gave her the most pleasure. It can be a trial and error in the beginning to find just the right ones.

Jo enjoyed our imaginative journeys to the mountains and to the ocean shore. Although we played two of our favorites, many times, she still seemed to reap the benefits from them and never grew tired of them. I noticed the benefits of each session almost immediately. Her face was more relaxed, her eyes brighter and she seemed calmer and ready to proceed with other activities at the conclusion of the imagery. Most importantly, she said that her pain was gone or diminished. I also benefited

from these sessions, coming out of them rested and revitalized. What I noticed after each session was that the atmosphere was altered in the room. It seemed calmer and more relaxed. The shared experience also created an atmosphere of intimacy between us that was very special. Sometimes, we talked for a few moments together sharing our journeys. Often, when I asked Jo how she enjoyed the session. She would respond, "It is really nice to be by myself."

Although, considered an alternative therapeutic technique, guided imagery has been used in psychotherapy for over a century. The documented use of guided imagery as a healing tool appears in all parts of the world: Asia, Australia, the Americas and Europe. Even Aristotle, Hippocrates and Galen utilized imagination and dream content for healing purposes. In 1985, Jeanne Achterberg wrote a book called Imagery in Healing, which is a classic in the alternative medicine field. It was very influential in promoting research into the practice of imagery by early healers and its effect on health promotion.

Since that time, there have been many clinical studies have been conducted on guided imagery that include hospitals, psychologists, the Mayo Clinic, the American Cancer Society and others. Clinical studies show the effectiveness of guided imagery to lower blood pressure and cholesterol and glucose levels in the blood. All these studies support the fact that the mind is a powerful ally in the healing process and can direct the body to make positive changes, even at a cellular level.

Whatever the mind thinks, the body manifests. An example would be if you imagined yourself running down a road while laying on a coach. Parts of the brain will send messages to the muscles that are involved in pre-motor activity, even though you are lying still. Golfers and other sport professionals practice their technique for the same reason. The body "sees" itself performing the activity due to the messages of the brain. It believes that what it "sees" is real and responds accordingly.

The Academy of Guided Imagery describes guided imagery as,

> ... a wide variety of techniques, including simple visualization and direct suggestion using imagery, metaphor and story-telling, fantasy exploration and game playing, dream interpretation, drawing, and active imagination where elements of the unconscious are invited to appear as images that can communicate with the conscious mind. [1]

The body tends to respond to mental imagery exactly as it would to a genuine external experience. During a guided imagery session, the senses, along with the body, are stimulated. It is both effective and enjoyable. Professionals in sports, business and other fields, who are aware of its effectiveness to effect change, have used imagery techniques to imagine themselves in a situation or with an ability that they want to achieve.

Guided imagery or thinking in images, is a right brained activity and it can influence other areas of the right hemisphere that include intuition, empathy, compassion, emotion, laughter and sensitivity to music. The more detailed the guided imagery, the more effective and the more personal the experience will

be. When attentive and relaxed, the listener is mentally transported to a serene and tranquil scene of his or her own design. Even though the script might suggest scenes such as a seashore, mountain meadow or a forested path, the listener invents the imagery from their own imagination.

Guided imagery is safe and simple to use and one can create their own imagery script, listen to recordings or experience a live session with a practitioner. It is a tool anyone can use. It is very cost effective for the benefits it delivers.

The Mayo Clinic states guided imagery provides the following benefits to clients:

1. Reduces the negative side effects of cancer treatments such as nausea, depression and fatigue.

2. Reduces pre-surgery fear and anxiety.

3. Reduces the need for prolonged pain medication and allows clients to leave hospital quicker.

4. Improves the client's ability to manage stress.

5. Reduces the severity of migraine headaches just as effectively as taking preventative medications.[2]

Besides the physiological and psychological benefits, guided imagery can also help with cognitive and behavioral issues. Guided imagery can mobilize unconscious processes to assist with conscious goals. You can use it to prepare for an athletic event, public performance or even a job interview. Through relaxed mental and physical states, positive suggestions can lead to the focusing and visualizing of goals. Creativity, healing and learning can take place easier in this transformative state.

GUIDED IMAGERY GUIDELINES

As with every practice, there are good ones and not so good one. Here are some guidelines that I found helpful when I selected a guided imagery script for Jo and for myself. The same guidelines are used if you are creating your own script.

First, you want to determine the goal of the imagery session. Is it for relaxation, pain management or is the purpose to stimulate creativity and motivation? Knowing the intention will help guide you to selecting the appropriate reading. Next, there needs to be an introduction to the session. This usually involves taking a few moments to prepare the body for relaxation (getting into a comfortable position and practicing some deep, cleansing breaths).

A guided "transition" will take the listener from their present state to one of deeper relaxation. There are different techniques used but the most commonly used one is that of a "countdown." Usually, the countdown begins with the number ten, the current state of the listener, and it descends to number one, being the most relaxed state. It is important that the countdown is spoken calmly and slowly, giving the listen time to relax further with each step. An example of such a countdown might sound like this:

We will count down from 10 and with each decreasing number; you will find yourself slipping deeper and deeper into a relaxed state. Let us begin...10...you are beginning to relax...9...8...you are relaxing more...7...6...you are becoming more and more relaxed....5...4... feel your body relax into complete comfort...3...you are feeling relaxed...2...1...you are now completely relaxed and feeling at peace.

It is common for guided imagery to lead the listener to peaceful place such as a forest path, mountaintop and seashore. A castle, cabin, cave, garden or a wildflower meadow can all work equally as well. The destination is limited only by imagination. After the listener has arrived at their "special place", they should be assured that they are safe and that they can take all the time they need to relax there.

A good guided imagery will encourage the listener to use all their senses to create and experience the journey. Include questions like, what colors do you see around you? Are there creatures nearby?" The more the details the listener can evoke, the more interactive the experience. It is also important that each stage of the journey provide the listener with enough time to really "be there," and that the suggestions are not delivered in rapid-fire speed! There should be plenty of appropriate pauses and rest breaks placed throughout the script.

After a certain time, the listener is told to return to their present state and leave their imagined environment. Sometimes they are asked to return to a starting point, such as a gate, doorway or path, which can also serve as their departure point. A good guided imagery will accomplish this departure slowly, encouraging a gentle awakening back to the room, rather than a rushed one. A "count up" will create a gentle transition back to the fully awakened state, starting at one this time and working up to ten. Once ten counts are reached, the listener will be asked to open their eyes and slowly adjust to their surroundings, taking all the time they need.

Here is an example of a guided imagery script:

In The Garden

We are going to journey to a place in nature where you can connect to a world of stillness and peace. It will be a relaxing and pleasant experience.

Put aside any worries or tension you may have and allow yourself to relax by taking a deep breath and then slowly release it....relax your body so that it is comfortable....close your eyes and let your face soften...let your jaw soften and relax...feel your shoulders drop.... Take a deep relaxing breath and feel your lungs completely..... As you slowly exhale, release any tension in your body ....Take another deep breath filling your lungs....exhale any remaining tension....feel yourself relax deeper....Feel yourself letting go of everything.

We will count down from 10 and with each decreasing number you will find yourself slipping deeper and deeper into a relaxed state. Let us begin...10...you are beginning to relax...9...8...you are relaxing more...7...6...you are becoming more and more relaxed....5...4... feel your body relaxing into complete comfort...3...you are feeling relaxed...2...1...you are now completely relaxed and feeling at peace.

You feel very calm and relaxed as you begin to look around you. You find you are on a path surrounded by meadows filled with colorful wildflowers ...take a moment to look at the flowers you see...What colors are they? What shapes are they? Take a moment to inhale the scented air. What does it smell like? Is it sweet or spicy? Notice how the brightness and fragrance of the flowers fills this place with freshness and delight.

As you walk down the path experience yourself connecting to the natural world around you...feel the warm, soft earth radiating beneath your feet....traveling up your body and soothing all your muscles and bones.... melting all tension away....You are becoming very light....very relaxed...very calm ....In the distance you see a garden and you begin to walk towards it slowly, enjoying the flowers, the scents and the birds singing in the trees as you go by. Soon you reach the garden and find it overflowing with flowers of every kind and color. Red orange, yellow, white, pink and blue blossoms everywhere....in the middle of the garden there is a large tree covered with bright yellow fruit....you sit beneath the tree, with your back against its trunk. You feel peaceful and happy at this place. Take a

moment to enjoy your surroundings.... As you sit there, you feel yourself slipping into a deeper relaxation. You look up through the branches of the tree at the sky and see the clouds float by. Let their shapes capture your imagination. Are there insects buzzing around you? Are there butterflies landing on the colorful flowers? Are there friendly creatures nearby? Maybe there are squirrels scampering across the branches....or hummingbirds flittering by....Notice the colors, patterns, scents and sounds that surround you in this beautiful place.... You can hear the birds singing in the trees. Take a moment to feel the beauty of this place and enjoy how bright and light everything is.

Soon you begin to notice a sweet, fresh scent coming from the golden fruits on the tree. They shimmer in the sunlight. You reach up and pick a fruit....it is light and slightly warm ....you watch it glow brightly in your palm....it feels like magic....so you take a bite of the fruit....and find that it is moist and delicious with a slight lemony taste. You feel the juice of this fruit warming your throat and filling your insides with a light. You take another bite and feel the light inside you growing stronger.... expanding....becoming brighter and brighter until you glow as bright as the sun. You feel fresh....light and joyful...full of energy and hope....you are radiating from every pore of your body and the garden reflects back your golden light. Enjoy this moment and all its gifts of health and radiance. You can stay in this relaxed state as long as you like knowing that you can always come back to this garden and the golden fruit tree whenever you want. Allow yourself to enjoy the golden light that envelops you. When you are ready to leave, give yourself a few minutes to gently return to the room and then open your eyes.

After a guided imagery or mindfulness meditation session you can offer your client an opportunity to journal about their experience.

POSITIVE AFFIRMATIONS

An affirmation is a positive statement about oneself or one's circumstances. It is phrased as if the statement is already true. It is the opposite of negative self-talk that so many of us do consciously and subconsciously. Jo showed me how important daily positive affirmations are when she said,

"That is good for me to hear. I need to hear those words every day."

Jo's gentle compassion towards others was one of her most endearing traits. Unfortunately, she did not always extend that compassion towards herself. I had to remind her that she had to have the same patience and acceptance of her limitations that she gave to others. She had been a loving mother to her two adult children but now at this time of her life, she had to be a nurturing mother to herself! I would encourage her not to say anything negative about herself, like such as "I am stupid or I am worthless."

This negative self-talk may at first seem innocent, but repeated enough times, over a course of years, works against us. Every thought we have about ourselves, when repeated often enough will become a belief system. Often negative self-talk takes the upper hand as it did in the case of Jo. The best way to turn this negative self-chatter around is not to say anything about yourself that you would not say to anyone else. Instead of focusing on the negative, focus on the positive and what is working well. Think about the things that you are thankful for in your life.

During her career as a professional geriatric nurse, she consistently gave others encouragement and hope. Now she would need to do the same for herself. I would often ask her what advice she would tell a young child or one of her patients if they came to her feeling hopeless and helpless. Would she tell them to give up or keep trying? Jo usually responded that she would encourage them. I would then explain that she would have to do the same--- learn how to ignore the negative thoughts that entered her mind when she thought about her recovery progress. It would be necessary to replace those negative thoughts with a positive statement that would help her stay focused on what was positive in her life.

EXERCISE: Positive Affirmations

Directions:

1. Have your client think of several things that they are thankful for in their lives or in goals they want to achieve. Write down these affirmations. Written positive affirmations are one of the most popular positive thinking exercises. Some examples of affirmations that Jo and I used were:

- Every day I am becoming stronger and healthier.

- My exercises are making me stronger.

- I am more relaxed and focused.

- I feel appreciative and grateful for everything in my life.

- I will motivate myself to exercise.

- My voice is getting stronger.

- I am strong!

- I am writing better.

- I am surrounded by people who love and care about me.

2. Decorate affirmations on index cards or whatever size paper works best. Use colorful markers to write the words. You and your client can design artwork to put with the words. Look in magazines for images that support the words and make a mini collage. Use glitter or stickers if you want. Have fun with this exercise.

3. Place the affirmation in a spot that your client can see every day. There are inexpensive magnetized plastic holders that the card can slip into at a craft store so it can hang on the refrigerator.

Post positive affirmations in a place where your client can see and read them every day. This will help them remember the affirmation.

Find an image to support that affirmation.

Take a few minutes before each session to read the affirmations aloud together.

Affirmation cards can also be found in gift stores and online.

Meditation

Meditation, a state of "thoughtless awareness," allows one to focus on the present moment rather than the past or future. The meditator concentrates on his or her own breath in its entirety and allows thoughts to pass through their mind without attachment or concern. Meditation trains the mind to become still and observing. Meditation trains us to sit undisturbed and relaxed in our body and allows us an opportunity to "attend" to ourselves without judgement. It helps us become aware of the tension and muscular tightness that may be present in our bodies. It allows us to observe our thoughts and emotions without a need to respond or judge.

Meditation is a continuous cycle of being, accepting and letting go. First with our breath, then our bodies and finally with our thoughts. Mindful meditation can lead to inner balance and stability, physical relaxation, emotional calmness, openness to joy, and the ability to be "fully present." Mindfulness meditation can be a salve for our nervous system. While stress activates the "fight or flight" part of our nervous system, mindfulness meditation gives us an opportunity to give it a rest. Our heart rate decreases, our respiration slows and our blood pressure drops."

Advocates of mindfulness practice attest that it is an effective method for the treatment for stress, worry, lack of focus, relationship problems, addictions and more. Those that practice mindfulness on a regular basis finds that it leads them to feel a greater sense of wellbeing and peacefulness. They find that it helps them achieve greater focus, as well as a sense of increased creativity and vitality. Clinical studies are showing the same positive results. Researchers at the University of Massachusetts Medical School, found that 90% of meditation practitioners in a control group experienced significant reduction in anxiety and depression too.

Reported results from the Massachusetts General Hospital (MGH) study, Mindfulness-Based Stress Reduction (MBSR), showed positive effects on psychological well-being. The MBSR study showed changes in gray matter concentration in brain regions involved in learning and memory processes, emotion regulation, self-referential processing, and perspective taking. Britta Hölzel, PhD, first author of the paper and a research fellow at MGH and Giessen University in Germany states,

Other studies in different patient populations have shown that meditation can make significant improvements in a variety of symptoms, and we are now investigating the underlying mechanisms in the brain that facilitate this change. It is fascinating to see the brain's plasticity and that, by practicing meditation, we can play an active role in changing the brain and can increase our well-being and quality of life. [3]

Current research has found moderate evidence that mindfulness meditation can help reduce pain, anxiety and depression, and can cause an increase in grey matter. However, further studies still need to be done to document its efficacy for other physical, emotional or mental ailments. There are many books, classes, online sites, videos, etc. that you can use with your client if they wish to explore mindfulness meditation.

As I did not use mindful meditation with Jo, I cannot speak from personal experience on its benefits for stroke patients. The reason guided imagery was chosen over mindfulness meditation was because the imaginative guided imagery scripts gave Jo an immediate distraction from her pain by filling her mind with images. It seemed the best choice of the two techniques for that point in her recovery.

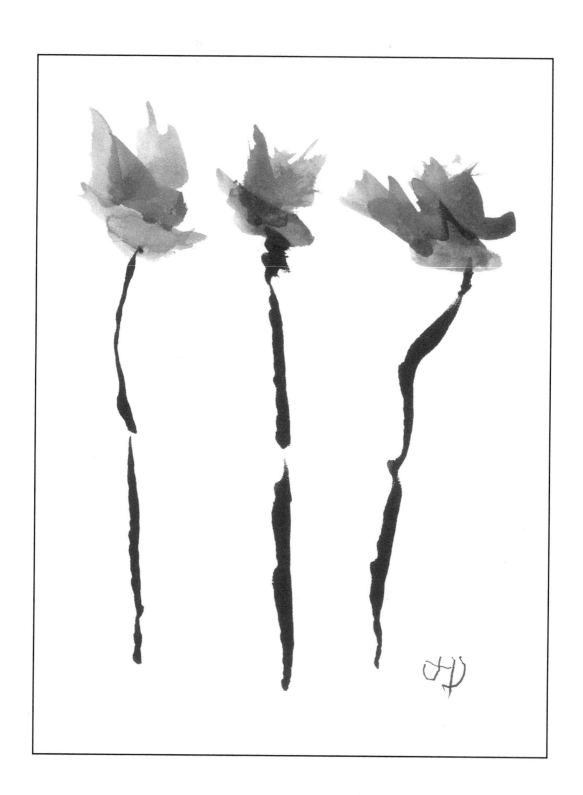

CHAPTER THIRTEEN

CONCLUSION

Jo demonstrated that a home cognitive recovery program that incorporates the creative arts could deliver effective results while still being enjoyable. By infusing the creative arts, Jo benefited from having a diverse range of learning experiences that were also stimulating. Jo's interest in the arts led to great improvement in her attention span. Over the years, Jo showed significant gains in memory, language, and executive thinking skills. She was able to control her non-dominant hand well enough to draw, paint, and play the keyboard. She also demonstrated awareness of her thought processes (metacognition) and was able to observe herself and initiate corrections in her activities. Many of these exercises were very challenging because she was developing several cognitive skills simultaneously.

Jo painted around fifty whimsical watercolors, many of which were displayed in the local art gallery, and all of which hang on her living room walls. Jo's artwork was her proudest accomplishment. The art activities provided many opportunities to exercise her cognitive skills. Jo's attention increased to where she could concentrate for more extended periods. Drawing, in particular, helped her to recognize patterns and understand the relationships between shapes, colors, and space. Jo's ability to process information visually and her eye, hand, and brain coordination improved over time.

Over the years, she began to show more initiative and creativity in her art as she blended colors of her choosing and drew playful figures and faces. I was excited when Jo began to observe herself as she painted or drew and could notice the mistakes she made. She then would attempt to correct them as best she could. At the end of an activity, Jo was able to communicate what she thought was successful, or what was not, about her painting. Best of all, doing art gave Jo a pleasurable distraction from her physical pain.

Music was another of our powerful cognitive activities we did. Research has shown that music can light up multiple areas of the brain and even help improve verbal memory. Its effects on Jo were amazing and immediate. I saw measurable progress in Jo's cognitive abilities: attention (ability to stay focused during the session), comprehension (learning new songs), memory (recalling several different songs), auditory processing (hearing the difference in notes), cognitive flexibly (ability to play the keyboard and sing) and metacognition (noticing and correcting her mistakes).

Playing music was a very kinesthetic activity. Jo learned how much pressure was needed for the keys and how to move her fingers up and down the keyboard. The coordination between Jo's eyes, hand, and brain were being strengthened, just like in the art activities. Jo's ability to process new information (learning a song or a new chord) and recall that information the next day was impressive. She could remember the songs we were doing. When Jo was first learning a song, the notes were printed on a music sheet and placed above the piano keys. She would refer to this as she played. When I felt she knew the song pretty well, I removed the music sheet and encouraged her to play by memory. Another cognitive challenged for her was to play the tune and sing at the same time. This proved very difficult, but occasionally, she was able to accomplish this.

Writing helped Jo work on her language skills. Writing activities included both the computer keyboard and the written journal. Both were excellent vehicles for her self-expression. Writing helped Jo improve her attention and concentration and provided opportunity to practice word recall and proper word usage. It also allowed her to work on eye, hand, and brain coordination. Best of all, it was another activity that Jo truly enjoyed, especially when she typed emails to family and friends. It helped widen her window on the world. Handwriting was a big struggle for her. There were days when her letters and words were good, and others when they were not. However, the mere act of attempting to write letters and form words was a good exercise for her brain. It integrates thinking, language, motor control, and visual processing skills.

Storytelling helped Jo improve cognitive and language building skills. I was hoping it would improve her auditory processing skills, and challenge her ability to recall and organize information. Jo demonstrated focused attention and understanding of read-aloud stories and enjoyed the activity very much. By reading a story aloud, Jo could hear the words and associate them with an image or meaning from memory. Story *writing offered the same cognitive stimulations as story reading, with the addition of elements of imagination, reasoning, and decision- making. Over the years, I helped Jo compose over eight short stories about her bird images. She enjoyed these activities very much.*

Guided imagery was added for relaxation. Whenever Jo was troubled with pain, we first attempted to relieve it through a guided imagery session. It had a very positive effect on Jo, and usually, pain diminished by the end of a 30- minute session. Practicing positive affirmations was a tool we used whenever Jo was feeling sad or depressed about her situation. This included listening to positive or inspirational videos about other people who have overcome obstacles in their lives. Both techniques were beneficial for her.

The more Jo practiced our cognitive exercises, the more improvement she showed in all her cognitive domains. Cognitive coaching is best when it is consistent. I saw some cognitive decline whenever our coaching sessions were interrupted for an extended period of time. Jo needed daily cognitive workouts or she would lose what she gained.

Remember that the journey to recovery will be different for everyone. The journey begins where the patient is at and continues from there. Every day will be different---it's a journey of ups, downs, and plateaus. The most important thing to remember is to never give up, and always work towards your goals!

Whatever You Can Do
Or Dream You Can Do,
Begin It.
Boldness Has Genius,
Power And Magic In It.
Begin It Now.

—GOETHE

EDUCATIONAL WEBSITES

Stroke Websites

American Stroke Association: www.strokeassociation.org

Canadian Stroke Association: canadianstrokenetwork.ca/en

European Stroke Organization: www.eso-stroke.org

National Stroke Association: www.stroke.org

North American Brain Injury Society: www.nabis.org

World Stroke Association: www.world-stroke.org

Caregiving Websites

Caregiver.Com: www.caregiver.com

Caring Com: www.caring.com

National Alliance for Caregiving: www.caregiving.org

Educational Websites

ABCYA: www.abcya.com

Education.com: www.education.com

Education World: www.educationworld.com

ESL Printables.com: www.eslprintables.com

Jump Start: www.jumpstart.com

K5 Learning: www.k5learning.com

Lesson Planet: www. lessonplanet.com

Phonic Talk: www.phonictalk.com

Puzzle Maker: www.puzzlemaker.discoveryeducation.com

Rhyme Zone: www.rhymezone.com

Soft Schools: www.softschools.com

Wordfinding.com: www.wordfinding.com

Word Search: www.thewordsearch.com

NOTES

Chapter Four

1. Boyatzis, Richard, Rochford, Kylie, Taylor, Scott, Front Psychol. 2015; 6: 670. *The role of the positive emotional attractor in shared vision toward effective leadership, relationships, and engagement.*

Chapter Five

1. Drucker, Peter. 1954. *The Practice of Management*, Harper, New York; Heinemann, London, 1955; revised ed., Butterworth-Heinemann, 2007.

Chapter Ten – Music

1. Sacks, O. W. 2007. *Musicophilia: Tales of music and the brain.* New York, N.Y.: Knopf.

2. Patel, A.D. 2008. *Music, language and the brain.* Oxford: Oxford University Press.

3. Schlaug G, Marchina S, Norton A. 2008. *From Singing to Speaking: Why Patients with Broca's Aphasia can sing and how that may lead to recovery of expressive language functions.* Music Perception 2008; 25:315-323.

4. Särkämö T, Tervaniemi M, Laitinen S, Forsblom A, Soinila S, Mikkonen M, Autti T, Silvennoinen HM, Erkkilä J, Laine M, Peretz I, Hietanen M. Brain. 2008 Mar;131(Pt 3):866-76. doi: 10.1093/brain/awn013.

5. Bittman, M.D., Barry. 2001."*Composite Effects of Group Drumming...,"Alternative Therapies in Health and Medicine;* Volume 7, No. 1, pp. 38-47.

6. Thaut, M.D., Michael. 2014. *"Handbook of Neurologic Music Therapy."* Oxford University Press.

7. Friedman,Robert Lawrence. 2000. *The Healing Power of the Drum.* White Cliffs Media Co.

8. Sacks. Ibid.

Chapter 12 – Guided Imagery

1. Achterberg, Jeanne. 2013. *Imagery in healing: Shamanism and modern medicine.* Shambhala Publications.

2. Hölzel, B. K., Lazar, S. W., Gard, T., Schuman-Olivier, Z., Vago, D. R., & Ott, U. 2011.

"How does mindfulness meditation work? Proposing mechanisms of action from a conceptual and neural perspective." Perspectives. *6*(6), 537-559.

3. Mayo Clinic. "Enhance Healing through Guided Imagery." ScienceDaily. ScienceDaily 7, January 2008.

BIBLIOGRAPHY

Adams, Kathleen. 1990. *Journal to the Self: 22 Paths to Personal Growth.* Warner Books, Inc. New York, NY.

Cameron, Julia. 1999. *Artist's Way: A Spiritual Path to Higher Creativity.* Penguin Random House. New York, NY.

Capacchione, Ph.D., Lucia. (2001). *The Power of Your Other Hand.* Career Press, Franklin Lakes, NY.

Campbell, Don G. 1997. *The Mozart Effect.* Avon Books, New York.

Edwards, Betty. 1989, 1999, 2012. *Drawing on the Right Side of the Brain.* Penguin Putnam. Seattle, WA.

Gardner, Howard. 2004. *Frames of Mind.* Basic Books. New York, NY.

Goleman, Daniel. 1995. *Emotional Intelligence.* Bantam Books, New York.

Hölzel, B. K., Lazar, S. W., Gard, T., Schuman-Olivier, Z., Vago, D. R., & Ott, U. (2011). How does mindfulness meditation work? Proposing mechanisms of action from a conceptual and neural perspective. *Perspectives on psychological science, 6*(6), 537-559.

Levine, Peter. 2018. *Stronger after Stroke: Your Roadmap to Recovery.* Spring Publishing Co., LLC, New York, NY.

Oech von, Roger. 1990. *A Whack on the Side of the Head: How You Can Be More Creative.* Warner Books. New York, NY.

Pennebaker, PhD., James, W. 1990. *Opening Up: The Healing Power of Expressing Emotions.* The Guildford Press. New York, NY.

Taylor Bolte, Jill. 2008. *My Stroke of Insight: A Brain Scientist's Personal Journey.* Viking Press. New York, NY.

Wooten, Victor. 2006. *The Music Lesson: A Spiritual Search for Growth through Music.* Penguin Group. New York, NY.

Yancoske, Kathleen, Gulick, Kristin. (2009). *Handwriting for Heroes: Learn to Write with Your Non-Dominant Hand in Six Weeks.* Loving Healing Press, Inc., Ann Arbor, MI.

CPSIA information can be obtained
at www.ICGtesting.com
Printed in the USA
FSHW020209280320
68558FS